Carb-Cycling Cookbook for Beginners

Elevate Your Fitness Journey with Carb-Cycling. Discover the Power of Strategic Carb Intake, Overcome Plateaus, and Revel in Delicious, Nutrient-Packed Recipes. Include 4 Week Meal Plan

By Mary Frow

Table of Contents

Introduction

The Evolution of Dieting and Where Carb-Cycling Fits

Dieting as a notion has been a part of human history for centuries, evolving in line with our understanding of nutrition, health, and the human body. Dieting is a reflection of our ever-changing relationship with food, our bodies, and our cultural expectations of health and beauty. From ancient societies' fasting practices to today's protein-packed diets, the terrain of dieting has been as diverse as it has been complex.

Dieting was never about losing weight or looking good. It was all about survival. Fasting was practiced by ancient civilizations such as the Greeks and Egyptians for religious and therapeutic causes. They believed that fasting might cleanse both the body and the spirit. This was a time when the relationship with food was primarily about subsistence and spiritual connection, rather than body image.

As nations advanced, so did their understanding of nutrition. The Renaissance period, for example, saw the growth of the notion in balancing physiological humors. Diets were suggested to preserve a balance between these humors and ensure good health. It was a primitive grasp of nutrition, but it was a start.

The twentieth century, on the other hand, saw a considerable transition. With the rise of mass media, societal standards of beauty grew more defined, and there was suddenly a global baseline for what was considered "ideal." This was the age of fad diets. From the cabbage soup diet to the grapefruit diet, people were looking for quick remedies to align themselves with these standards. It was an era of experimentation, with various diets promising quick results but frequently at the expense of long-term health.

In the middle of this tornado of eating trends, nutrition science began to take center stage. Researchers began to comprehend the complex link between food, metabolism, and general health. This was the beginning of diets based on scientific principles rather than simply trends. Carb-cycling arose from this context of increasing understanding.

Carb-cycling is really about harnessing the body's metabolic processes for maximum health and performance. Unlike many diets that offer a one-size-fits-all approach, carb-cycling acknowledges the dynamic character of our bodies. It recognizes that our dietary demands fluctuate depending on things such as activity level, hormone changes, and even everyday stressors.

So, where does carb-cycling fit into the broader scheme of dieting? It is a blend of traditional wisdom and modern science. Carbohydrate cycling, like fasting, comprises periods of reduced carbohydrate intake. However, it does so with a thorough understanding of modern nutritional research. It is not about denying the body, but rather about carefully fueling it. On some days, the body may benefit from a carbohydrate rush, particularly after vigorous physical exertion. On the other hand, it may flourish on lesser carbohydrate intake, allowing it to draw into fat stores for energy.

For newbies, especially those eager to begin their carb-cycling adventure, understanding this diet's place in the larger context is critical. It's not a passing fad, but rather an approach based on an awareness of our bodies' cycles and demands. It's about listening to our bodies, recognizing the signals they convey, and responding with the appropriate nutritional choices.

Furthermore, carb-cycling demonstrates that dieting is no longer solely about weight loss. It is all about overall well-being. It's all about energy, mental clarity, and long-term wellness. Carb-cycling stands out in an information-overloaded society where every new day appears to herald the advent of a new diet craze. It is not about dramatic measures or severe limits. It's about striking a balance, comprehending, and making informed decisions.

Carb-cycling is a light of hope for those who have often become lost in the maze of nutritional information, jumping from one diet to another in search of the illusive 'ideal' routine. It's a good reminder that the healthiest diet isn't about following strict rules, but about recognizing and honoring our body.

Carbohydrate cycling is a tribute to how far we've come in the enormous timeframe of nutritional evolution. Our history with diets has been lengthy and varied, ranging from primitive fasting rituals through modern metabolic understanding. And today, with the wisdom of the past and the understanding of the present, carb-cycling offers a promising road forward. A route that promises more than simply weight loss, but also a healthier, more balanced existence.

Setting the Stage: What to Expect from This Book

Starting a new diet can feel like you're standing on the rim of a huge, undiscovered land. The road ahead is unclear, full with potential obstacles, discoveries, and transformations. This sense of eagerness, mingled with apprehension, is natural. After all, the world of nutrition is huge, and the sheer number of available information can be intimidating. But what if there existed a guide, a compass, that could steer you through this complex environment, ensuring that every step you take is informed, confident, and in line with your objectives? This book is intended to be a guiding force for you.

Consider yourself an artist, with your body serving as the canvas. Every meal you eat, every dietary decision you make, is a brushstroke on this canvas. These brushstrokes combine to form a picture, which reflects your health, vigor, and well-being. However, in order to create a masterpiece, an artist must have the proper tools, skills, and, most importantly, knowledge. This book is intended to provide you with these necessities, ensuring that every brushstroke and food choice contributes to a healthier, more vibrant you.

For those unfamiliar with the concept of carb-cycling, you may be wondering, "Why this diet?" What distinguishes it from the plethora of other diets that have acquired popularity over the years? The solution is in its approach. Carbohydrate cycling is not about restriction or deprivation. It's about understanding your body's rhythm, the ebb and flow of its energy requirements, and adapting your diet to match. It's a dance, a ballet of nutrition and metabolism in which every step is calculated but flexible.

As you go deeper into these pages, you'll learn about the science of carb-cycling. But don't worry, this won't be a long, jargon-filled lecture. Instead, it will be a journey of discovery in which complicated concepts are reduced to little morsels of insight. You'll discover the role of carbs in our bodies and how they affect our energy levels, mood, and even weight. You'll debunk the fallacies that have long obscured our understanding of this critical macronutrient. Most importantly, you'll discover how to harness the power of carbs, using them as a tool to shape your body and improve your health.

But, as they say, knowledge is only potent when used. As a result, this book will go beyond simply conveying knowledge. It will provide you with useful tools, such as delicious, simple meals that adhere to carb-cycling principles. These dishes are designed with the novice in mind, whether they are new to the kitchen or the concept of carb-cycling. They are intended to be more than just meals; they are culinary experiences that satisfy not only the body but also the soul.

Why, in an age when information is just a click away, would one invest in a book? Recipes, diet programs, and nutritional advice abound on the internet. The problem is that not all information is created equal. While the digital age has been a godsend, it has also resulted in information overload. Every day, new diets are introduced, each claiming to be the 'ultimate' road to health and wellness. How does one tell fact from fiction in such a situation? How does one cut through the clutter and focus on what truly matters? This book is the culmination of extensive research, a distillation of scientifically supported principles, and years of practical experience. It's not simply a collection of recipes or diet recommendations; it's a comprehensive guide, a mentor who will accompany you on your carb-cycling adventure.

As you turn each page, you'll find stories and experiences that bring the ideas of carb-cycling to life. These testimonies attest to the transformational power of this diet. They are true stories of real people, people who, like you, were once on the brink of this unknown territory, fearful but hopeful. Their experiences, problems, and achievements will provide both motivation and insight, ensuring that you never feel alone on this journey.

This book is a companion as well as a guide. It serves as a link between where you are now and where you want to be. It's a tapestry of knowledge, practical tools, and inspiration stitched with care, competence, and a thorough grasp of your needs as a novice. As you embark on this trip, know that every obstacle you will face, every question you will have, and every desire you will have has been studied and handled in these pages.

As you lay the groundwork for this revolutionary journey, keep in mind that every great change begins with a single step. This book represents that first step, a leap of faith toward a healthier, more empowered you. Accept it with an open heart and an open mind, and watch as the magic of carb-cycling develops one delectable, informed, and creative brushstroke at a time.

Chapter 1: The Comprehensive Guide to Carbohydrates

Beginning a trip into the world of nutrition can feel like trying to find your way through a labyrinth. Advice, new insights, and opposing viewpoints emerge at every turn. Carbohydrates are one of the most contested and misunderstood parts of our diet despite the abundance of information available on the topic. Their genuine significance in our health and wellbeing has been glorified and condemned, leaving many of us confused.

This section is meant to serve as a guidepost, leading you through the maze of information surrounding carbohydrates. We'll get into the weeds, debunking myths and illuminating the science underlying these vital chemicals. We'll cover everything from carbs' biological function to their effect on our weight, so you can approach them with knowledge and certainty.

As we travel together, keep in mind that gaining insight is the cornerstone of personal agency. You'll be better able to make educated, well-rounded nutritional decisions if you have a firm grasp on carbs, their benefits, and their drawbacks. This chapter is full with helpful information that will improve your diet and lifestyle whether you're an experienced nutritionist or just getting started.

The Biology of Carbs: Simple vs. Complex

Carbohydrates are one of the most talked, contested, and frequently misunderstood components of our diet in the broad realm of nutrition. They've been both hated and celebrated, causing a tornado of confusion for many, particularly those just starting out on their path to understand nutrition. To really understand the function of carbohydrates in our diet and health, we must first investigate their biology, unlocking the mystery of simple vs complex carbohydrates.

Consider a bustling city for a moment. Roads, highways, and lanes symbolize the various paths in our bodies that digest food. Consider two sorts of vehicles on these roads: agile motorcycles that can maneuver through traffic quickly, and huge trucks that drive more deliberately while carrying greater loads. Simple carbs are analogous to these motorcycles, but complex carbs are analogous to the larger trucks.

Simple carbohydrates, which are commonly present in meals such as candy, pastries, and drinks, are molecularly simple. Consider them the basic units of energy, similar to those motorcycles flying through our bloodstream. When we ingest a sugary drink or a candy bar, our bodies do not have to work hard to digest it. The sugar enters our system quickly, causing a surge in energy. It's the thrill you get after drinking a sweetened beverage, a burst of energy. However, similar to the transitory nature of motorcycles speeding by, this energy surge is fleeting, often leading to an inevitable crash and a dramatic drop in energy levels.

Complex carbs, on the other hand, are the unsung heroes of long-term energy. They are molecularly more complex and can be found in foods such as whole grains, legumes, and vegetables. Consuming them is like to putting larger trucks on our city streets. Our bodies take their time, breaking them down piece by bit, extracting energy gradually and consistently. There is no quick rush or spike, but rather a constant release of vitality that keeps us running for a longer period of time. It's the difference between a sprint and a marathon, between a quick burst and sustained endurance.

But why is this distinction important, especially for someone new to carb-cycling or nutrition in general? The answer is in the effect these carbohydrates have on our bodies and general health. The quick energy boost from simple carbohydrates may feel exhilarating, but it is frequently accompanied by an increase in insulin, our body's way of managing blood sugar. Consistently elevated insulin levels can lead to a variety of health problems, ranging from weight gain to more serious illnesses like diabetes. It's similar to the wear and tear on roads caused by continual, high-speed motorcycle traffic, which causes potholes and degradation.

Complex carbohydrates, with their consistent energy delivery, promote a more balanced insulin response. They nourish our bodies without creating drastic hormonal changes. Furthermore, they include a plethora of other nutrients such as fiber, vitamins, and minerals, all of which help to our general health. Consuming them is analogous to maintaining our city streets, guaranteeing smooth traffic flow, and minimizing wear and tear.

Understanding this distinction is critical for newcomers, especially those eager to embrace carb-cycling. It is not only about measuring carbs, but also about determining the quality of these carbs. It's about making informed decisions, choosing foods that nourish and maintain rather than providing a quick fix. It's the foundation upon which the entire carb-cycling edifice is built.

Remember this distinction as you go on your culinary adventures, creating delectable low-carb meals. Choose whole grains instead of refined flours, fresh fruits instead of sweet liquids, and legumes instead of packaged treats. These decisions will determine the success of your carb-cycling trip, ensuring you maximize the benefits of this strong nutritional approach.

Carbohydrates, in all their various forms, play an important role in the magnificent tapestry of nutrition. They are the principal fuel source for our bodies, providing the energy that propels our daily activities. But, like with everything else in life, it's the quality that counts, not the number. Understanding carb biology, the dance of basic versus complicated, is more than just getting knowledge; it is about empowering yourself. One delicious, informed bite at a time, you're taking the first, critical step toward a healthier, more vibrant existence.

How the Body Processes and Uses Carbs

Carbohydrates play a vital and complex melody in the intricate symphony of our body's operations. Carbohydrates may appear to be basic dietary components to the uninformed, but they are the primary fuel that powers the very essence of our being. Uncovering the mysteries of an age-old dance, a rhythm that has sustained life for millennia, is analogous to unraveling the secrets of an age-old dance.

Consider a booming mill by a tranquil river. Water rushes through the mill, rotating the wheel and grinding grains into flour. In many ways, this mill resembles our body's complicated process of turning carbohydrates into energy. The river's flow reflects the carbohydrates we ingest, and the flour represents the energy that keeps us going. But how does this shift take place? How does our body transform a bowl of oats or a slice of bread into the vitality that propels our every movement?

Carbohydrates take an interesting journey through our bodies when we consume them. Enzymes like amylase begin the process of breaking down these complicated compounds in our mouth. As we chew, the carbs in our food begin to break down into simpler sugars, ready for the next stage of their journey.

These sugars move from the mouth to the stomach and then to the small intestine. They are further subdivided into their most fundamental forms here: glucose, fructose, and galactose. It's a laborious process that ensures these sugars are tiny enough to be absorbed by our bodies. Once absorbed, glucose, the main sugar, takes center stage.

Our blood, a vast highway that reaches every nook and cranny of our bodies, transports this glucose to every cell, providing much-needed fuel. However, its delivery is not random or chaotic. It's meticulously planned and controlled by the hormone insulin. Insulin, which is produced by our pancreas, functions as a gatekeeper, allowing glucose to enter our cells and be used as energy. It keeps our blood sugar levels steady, neither too high nor too low, preserving a vital balance for our health.

But what happens when our cells have had their fill, when they have gotten all the glucose they require? Is it true that extra glucose floats aimlessly in our bloodstream? Not exactly. In its infinite wisdom, our body has a system for storing this excess for future use. The liver and muscles convert glucose into glycogen, which serves as a reserve fuel. Consider it our body's savings account, a reserve of energy for times when we may want an extra boost, such as during intensive physical exercise or in between meals.

There is, however, a limit to how much glycogen our bodies can store. Once these reserves are depleted, any remaining glucose is transformed into fat, a long-term energy storage form. This mechanism guarantees that no energy source is wasted, and that every carbohydrate we take is either used immediately, stored for short-term use, or preserved for later use.

This understanding is critical for anyone new to the realm of nutrition, especially those interested in carb-cycling. It explains why the timing and kind of carbs are important. Consuming simple carbs, which are quickly broken down, can cause rapid rises in blood sugar, resulting in an insulin surge. If this pattern persists, our bodies may fail to balance blood sugar efficiently, leading to a variety of health issues. Complex carbohydrates, on the other hand, provide a continuous release of glucose, delivering sustained energy without abrupt increases.

Understanding how our bodies store extra glucose allows us to comprehend the significance of balancing carb intake with physical exercise. What about our glycogen reserves in the liver and muscles? They are activated during exercise, ensuring that our bodies get the fuel they require to work optimally. It's a delicate balance that carb-cycling seeks to optimize by ensuring that we ingest carbs when our bodies require them and cut back when they don't.

Carbohydrates are more than just a nutritional component; they are evidence of our body's remarkable ability to collect, absorb, and utilize energy. Every grain, fruit, and vegetable we eat starts a chain reaction, a dance of hormones, enzymes, and cells all working together to power the very essence of life. Remember this dance, this beat as you dig deeper into the world of carb-cycling. Allow it to direct your choices, enlighten your decisions, and inspire you on your road to a better, more vibrant you.

Debunking Myths: Carbs and Weight Gain

Few topics in the ever-changing world of nutrition have been as highly disputed and misunderstood as the function of carbs in weight gain. Carbohydrates have been hailed as crucial energy sources in one age and demonized as waistline-expanding villains in the next, with the narrative shifting over time. These contradictory messages can be both perplexing and daunting for someone who is just starting out in the world of nutrition and carb-cycling. It's past time to clear the air, debunking fallacies and clarifying the genuine relationship between carbs and body weight.

Let's start with one of the most common misconceptions: "Eating carbs will make you fat." In its simplistic form, this statement has led many people to avoid carbohydrates totally, fearing their potential impact on the scale. The reality, however, is significantly more nuanced. Carbohydrates, by themselves, are not the cause of undesirable weight gain. The kind, quantity, and total caloric intake, as well as individual exercise levels, dictate how carbs affect our weight.

Consider a beautiful, quiet lake with calm, pure water. Consider a stream that flows into this lake. The lake level remains steady if the water pouring in equals the water draining out. However, if more water flows in than flows out, the lake begins to overflow. Our bodies follow a similar logic. Like the water flowing into the lake, the food we eat gives calories. Our activities, from walking to thinking, expend calories, which resemble the water flowing out. When we consume more calories than we burn, regardless of whether they come from carbohydrates, fats, or proteins, our bodies retain the excess, resulting in weight gain.

Another popular misconception is that "all carbs are created equal." Nothing could be further from the truth. As previously discussed, there is a world of difference between simple and complex carbs. While simple carbs, such as those found in sugary snacks and drinks, can cause rapid blood sugar spikes and subsequent crashes, complex carbs, such as those found in whole grains and vegetables, provide continuous energy. Overreliance on the former can lead to overeating as the body wants additional nutrition after the initial energy boost wears off. Meals high in complex carbohydrates, on the other hand, keep us content for longer, lowering the probability of overconsumption.

There's also the misconception that "carbs are empty calories." This viewpoint depicts carbohydrates in broad strokes, omitting the plethora of vital elements they can give. Whole grains are high in fiber, which aids digestion and promotes heart health. Fruits are high in vitamins, minerals, and antioxidants, all of which contribute to our general health. Labeling such nutrient-dense foods as "empty" is not only deceptive, but also detrimental to individuals seeking a balanced, holistic approach to nutrition.

For individuals considering carb-cycling, it's critical to approach carbs with an open mind, free of the constraints of these beliefs. Carbohydrates are not the enemy; unbalance is. We may enjoy the benefits of carbohydrates without the dreaded weight gain if we understand how to harness their power and line their intake with our bodies' demands. Listening to our bodies, acknowledging the signals they provide, and responding with informed, conscious decisions are all part of the process.

Myths and misconceptions are sure to emerge in the enormous tapestry of nutrition advice. They spread, establishing themselves in our collective awareness and influencing our beliefs and habits. However, knowledge is power. We empower ourselves to make decisions that match with our particular needs and aspirations by discovering the truth and challenging widely accepted beliefs. Carbohydrates, like any other nutrient in our diet, have a place. They are neither good nor bad essentially. The way we assimilate them, the decisions we make on a daily basis, affects their impact on our health and weight.

Remember to consider carbs as allies, not foes, as you dig deeper into carb-cycling, armed with recipes and insights. They are an important element of our dietary landscape because they provide energy, minerals, and flavors. You're reclaiming the narrative, writing your own tale of health, balance, and well-being by knowing them and refuting the myths that surround them.

Chapter 2: Diving Deep into Carb-Cycling

The word "carb-cycling" may sound mysterious to the uninformed, but it actually refers to a profoundly transformative journey. It's more than simply a way of eating; it's a way of life, a symphony in perfect harmony with our evolutionary past. This chapter will delve deeply into carb-cycling, covering its history, the science behind it, and the many advantages it provides. Carb-cycling is a symphony of health on all levels, from the physical to the mental and from the concrete to the abstract. Carb-cycling, as we set out on this journey, is about more than simply the food we eat; it's about the way we live, the vitality we exude, and the clarity with which we approach the world.

The Origins and Science Behind Carb-Cycling

Few tactics in the vast world of nutrition have captivated the imagination and interest of fitness enthusiasts and health-conscious consumers as carb-cycling has. But where did this idea come from? And what is the science behind its principles? To properly grasp carb-cycling's strength and potential, we must first go back to its origins and delve deeply into the mechanics that make it so powerful.

The history of carbohydrate cycling is connected with the history of dietary practices aimed at optimizing human performance. Athletes, particularly endurance runners and bodybuilders, were intuitively adjusting their carbohydrate intake long before the word "carb-cycling" entered our vernacular. They discovered that carbohydrate eating timing and amount could affect energy levels, muscle recovery, and overall performance. This empirical knowledge, derived from countless hours of training and observation, established the framework for carb-cycling, which was eventually institutionalized.

However, it wasn't until the late twentieth century that scientists became interested in the metabolic implications of varied carbohydrate intake. The researchers discovered that switching between periods of high and low carbohydrate consumption had a significant impact on how the body used energy. On high-carb days, the body would primarily burn glucose, which was acquired from the carbs consumed, whereas on low-carb days, the body would shift to using stored fat for fuel. This oscillation between metabolic states offered an enticing opportunity: Could this process be used to enhance fat loss and muscle growth?

The physiological basis of carb-cycling became clearer as the scientific investigation progressed. The hormone insulin is at the heart of this method. Carbohydrates are broken down into glucose, which enters the circulation when we consume them. In reaction, the pancreas secretes insulin, which aids in the transport of glucose into cells for utilization as energy. Insulin levels rise on high-carb days, boosting muscle glycogen storage and providing enough energy for high-intensity activities. On low-carb days, insulin levels remain low, prompting the body to use its fat reserves for fuel.

This dance between glucose and insulin is more than a metabolic process; it's a finely tuned symphony that determines whether we burn or store fat. One can theoretically direct this symphony by judiciously cycling carbohydrate intake, orchestrating periods of fat burning and muscle development.

However, carb-cycling science isn't only about insulin and glucose. It is also about adaptability. The human body is remarkable in its ability to adapt to dietary and environmental changes. When the body is treated to a constant low-carb diet, it becomes more efficient at fat oxidation, improving its ability to use fat as a primary energy source. This state, known as metabolic flexibility, is essential for carbohydrate cycling. It guarantees that the body can switch between fuel sources effortlessly, optimizing energy consumption based on dietary intake and physical demands.

But what about the brain, which is largely a glucose-dependent organ? Another unique aspect of carb-cycling can be found here. The liver begins to create ketones, an alternative fuel derived from fat, during extended low-carb periods. In the absence of adequate glucose, these ketones can pass the blood-brain barrier, providing an essential energy source for the brain. This ability to make and use ketones highlights the body's extraordinary adaptability as well as the potential benefits of carb-cycling.

It's critical to approach the complexities of carb-cycling with a feeling of wonder and inquiry. Here's an approach based on both old knowledge and modern science that promises to improve our health and performance by harnessing our bodies' intrinsic metabolic system. It demonstrates the human body's plasticity, resilience, and persistent will to optimize and thrive. As you begin your carb-cycling journey, keep in mind that you are taking part in a rich tapestry of human exploration, one that tries to understand and harness the very essence of our metabolic being.

Physiological Benefits: Beyond Just Weight Loss

In our current world, where the attraction of quick cures and instant gratification frequently trumps deeper understanding, it's easy to dismiss carb-cycling as merely a weight-loss method. However, doing so would be missing the forest for the trees. Carbohydrate cycling, with its rhythmic dance between high and low carbohydrate days, provides a slew of physiological benefits that go far beyond the weighing scale. Let's go on a journey to discover these numerous advantages, investigating how carb-cycling can have a significant impact on our general health and well-being.

The concept of metabolic flexibility is central to carb-cycling. While it may sound like a phrase from a science fiction novel, this term is firmly entrenched in our evolutionary history. Our forefathers had to adapt to shifting food supplies because they did not have the luxury of continuous meals. There were periods when fruits, tubers, and possibly the rewards of a good hunt were plentiful. But there were also hard periods when food was scarce. In its infinite wisdom, the human body developed to accommodate these oscillations, creating the ability to effortlessly transition between burning carbohydrates and fats for energy. This adaptability is the result of metabolic flexibility in action. By embracing carb-cycling, we tap into an old process, educating our bodies to be efficient fat burners while still utilizing carbohydrates for energy when available.

But how does this affect our overall health? For instance, greater blood sugar management has been linked to increased metabolic flexibility. As the body relies more on fat for energy on low-carb days, it becomes more sensitive to insulin, the hormone responsible for transporting glucose into cells. This increased insulin sensitivity can be beneficial, especially in a society where insulin resistance and type 2 diabetes are on the rise. By allowing our bodies to rest from constant carbohydrate assault, we allow our metabolic mechanism to reset, promoting better glucose regulation.

There's also the issue of inflammation. Chronic inflammation, termed the "silent killer," has been linked to a wide range of modern diseases, from heart disease to autoimmune disorders. According to new research, carb-cycling, particularly the low-carb phases, may have anti-inflammatory effects. The body produces fewer insulin spikes during these stages, which can limit the release of pro-inflammatory chemicals. Furthermore, it has been demonstrated that the formation of ketones, particularly beta-hydroxybutyrate, during prolonged low-carb periods has anti-inflammatory characteristics. Thus, by embracing the ebb and flow of carb-cycling, we may be arming our bodies with a powerful anti-inflammatory tool.

Carbohydrate cycling can boost brain function in addition to lowering blood sugar and inflammation. The brain, a voracious energy user, has long been thought to be predominantly reliant on glucose. Recent discoveries, however, have shed light on the brain's potential to use other fuel sources, particularly ketones. The liver creates ketones during periods of low carbohydrate intake when the body depletes its fat reserves. These chemicals, which were previously assumed to be a consequence of fat metabolism, are now recognized as a powerful brain fuel. They have been proven to increase brain energy generation, decrease oxidative stress, and even promote the formation of new synaptic connections. Those who engage in carb-cycling may benefit from enhanced cognitive function, sharper attention, and possibly even protection against neurodegenerative disorders.

Let me discuss a benefit that, while maybe intangible, is no less important: resilience. We're not simply optimizing metabolism when we subject our bodies to the rhythmic changes of carb-cycling; we're also creating resilience. We're teaching our bodies to thrive in the face of change, to find balance in the midst of chaos. This adaptability, this ability to ebb and flow with changing conditions, demonstrates the human body's intrinsic desire to thrive rather than just survive.

While weight loss may be the siren song that lures many people to carbohydrate cycling, the genuine magic lies under the surface. Carbohydrate cycling provides a symphony of advantages that resonate with the very essence of our physiological being, from metabolic flexibility to brain health, from inflammation control to promoting resilience. As you progress down this path, keep in mind that each high and low-carb day is a stride toward holistic well-being, a dance with our evolutionary heritage, and a celebration of the human body's limitless potential.

Psychological Benefits: Energy, Mood, and Mental Clarity

The carb-cycling journey is more than just a physical one. While the physical effects are significant, the psychological landscape it creates is equally transformational. We're not simply fueling our muscles and organs as we navigate the undulating terrains of high and low-carb days; we're also sustaining our thoughts, moods, and spirits. Let's look at the significant psychological benefits of carb-cycling, and how this nutritional approach may be a source of energy, mood elevation, and crystalline mental clarity.

Life's currency is energy. It's the pulsing energy that runs through our blood, propelling us through our days with zest and zeal. Traditional diets, with their steady input of carbohydrates, frequently result in energy swings. The highs are exhilarating, but the crashes may be crippling. With its cyclic modulation, carb-cycling provides a more harmonious energy landscape. The body enjoys the rapid energy that carbs deliver on high-carb days. Low-carb days result in a consistent, prolonged release of energy when the body delves into its fat reserves. This energy is not only physical, but also mental and emotional. It's the kind of vitality that not only gets you through the day, but makes it worthwhile to live.

Mood goes hand in hand with energy. Our emotional health is inextricably linked to our eating choices. The nutrients we feed the brain, that complicated organ of cognition and emotion, have a significant impact on it. Carb-cycling can help to stabilize mood by establishing a balance of immediate and prolonged energy sources. On low-carb days, the consistent energy from fat metabolism can help to prevent the emotional swings that commonly accompany energy crashes. Furthermore, ketones have been related to the release of neurotransmitters such as GABA, which has a soothing, mood-stabilizing impact. Thus, carb-cycling can be a source of emotional stability in a world fraught with mood swings.

However, the psychological fabric of carb-cycling extends beyond energy and mood to brain clarity. In the cacophony of modern life, with its never-ending flood of stimuli, mental clarity is a prized possession. It is the ability to see through the fog and navigate problems with clarity of thought. Carb-cycling, especially during low-carb phases, can be an effective tool in this quest. When the body creates ketones, these molecules nourish the brain as well as the muscles. Ketones have been demonstrated in studies to increase cognitive performance, minimize brain fog, and even improve memory. We're not simply feeding our bodies when we embrace carb-cycling; we're also strengthening our thoughts.

Carb-cycling's psychological effects are essentially a symphony of energy, mood stabilization, and brain clarity. It's a dance of the mind and spirit, a celebration of the human psyche's limitless possibilities. Remember that as you go through the ups and downs of carb-cycling, you're molding your soul as well as your body.

Chapter 3: The Mechanics of Carb-Cycling

Carb-cycling is like setting sail on a large ocean, where the waves reflect the highs and lows of carb intake and the horizon represents the goals one hopes to reach. "The Mechanics of Carb-Cycling," Chapter 3, acts as your compass, guiding you through the complexities of this dietary approach. After delving into the fundamentals of carbs and their critical function in our diet, this chapter will peel back the layers to reveal the 'how-tos' of carb-cycling. We'll traverse the waters of carb-cycling with precision and clarity, from knowing the strategic timing of carb intake to the interplay of proteins and fats in this regimen. This chapter promises to be a beacon, illuminating the route and providing an informed, effective, and transforming trip for every beginning embarking on this journey.

Mapping Out High-Carb and Low-Carb Days

Beginning the carb-cycling voyage is like to setting sail on the enormous ocean of nutritional knowledge. The waves rise and fall, the tides ebb and flow, and one discovers a harmonious equilibrium that resonates with the body's inner understanding in the midst of this rhythmic dance. The art of planning high-carb and low-carb days is key to this journey. It's not just about counting carbs or according to a strict regimen; it's about recognizing your body's requirements, listening to its murmurs, and charting a route that corresponds to its natural cycles.

Consider the body to be a huge symphony for a time. Every instrument, from the delicate flute to the strong drums, is important. Carbohydrates are like the powerful pulses of the percussion section in this symphony. The drums play a fast, exhilarating tune on high-carb days, providing immediate energy, replenishing glycogen stores, and supporting intense physical activities. These are the days when the body rejoices in the excess of glucose, which serves as the major fuel for our muscles and brain. It's a day to celebrate vitality, when the body is primed for activities like weight training, running, or any effort that necessitates short bursts of high energy.

Low-carb days, on the other hand, are like the smooth, calming tones of a violin. The energy is more muted and long-lasting. Instead of relying on carbohydrates for immediate energy, the body delves into its fat reserves and burns them for fuel. It provides a slower, more prolonged supply of energy, making it excellent for activities such as lengthy walks, yoga, or simply getting through one's daily routine. The body reaches a state of metabolic flexibility on these days, smoothly moving between carbs and fats for energy. It demonstrates the body's plasticity, its ability to establish equilibrium in the always shifting environment of our food choices.

How does one go about mapping these high and low-carb days, one would wonder? The beauty of carb-cycling is its adaptability. There is no one-size-fits-all solution. It is instead a matter of tuning into the body's demands and adjusting accordingly. High-carb days may coincide with the most challenging workouts for someone who engages in severe physical training, ensuring that the muscles have enough fuel to operate at their best. For someone who is more inactive, the high-carb days could be spaced out more, giving the body more time to draw into its fat reserves.

The trick is to pay attention, observe, and adjust. Begin with a basic framework, such as rotating between high and low carb days, and then fine-tune based on how your body responds. Do high-carb days make you feel energized and vibrant? Or are you lethargic and bloated? What about the carb-free days? Do you feel light and clear-headed, or exhausted and foggy? These are the body's whispers, the subtle indications that steer the carb-cycling path.

It's also important to understand that carbohydrate cycling isn't about deprivation. It's not about eliminating carbs or demonizing them. Carbohydrates are a crucial part of our diet, supplying necessary nutrients and energy in their natural, unprocessed form. On high-carb days, enjoy the pleasure of biting into a luscious fruit, the comfort of a bowl of oatmeal, and the energy that these meals provide. On low-carb days, enjoy the satiation provided by healthy fats, the sustained energy provided by proteins, and the diverse flavors of non-starchy veggies.

Planning high-carb and low-carb days is an experiment, a balancing act between abundance and restriction. It's a process of discovery, of knowing one's own body's cycles, and of striking a balance that works for one's specific requirements and goals. Remember that carb-cycling is not a rigorous regimen; rather, it is a fluid, adaptable strategy that honors the body's knowledge and ability to find harmony among the ebb and flow of our dietary choices.

The Role of Protein and Fats in Carb-Cycling

Proteins and lipids weave intricate patterns of sustenance and endurance in the broad tapestry of nutrition, where carbs paint brilliant strokes of immediate energy. As we learn more about the physics of carb-cycling, it becomes clear that this nutritional approach is about more than just the ebb and flow of carbohydrates. It's a symphonic symphony in which proteins and fats play key roles in complementing the carbohydrate dance and ensuring that the body remains nourished, balanced, and poised for peak performance.

Consider a typical day in your life. The sun rises, providing a golden color, and you begin your high-carb day. Carbohydrates provide energy for your immediate tasks, such as a morning run or an intense training session. However, as the day goes, proteins and fats take center stage, ensuring that your energy does not dwindle, your muscles repair, and your body remains full.

Proteins, frequently referred to as the "building blocks of life," serve a variety of roles in carbohydrate cycling. They repair and develop tissues at the cellular level, making them vital for persons who exercise. After a hard workout, when the muscles are like sponges eager to absorb nutrition, it is the proteins that step in, healing the wear and tear and stimulating muscle growth. However, their function is not restricted to muscle restoration. Proteins also produce enzymes, hormones, and other substances, which ensure that the body's biochemical reactions run smoothly. They give a consistent source of energy, especially on low-carb days, guaranteeing that the body does not feel starved or drained of energy.

Then there are lipids, which are frequently misunderstood and unfairly demonized in the field of nutrition. Fats emerge as unsung heroes in the world of carb-cycling. When carbs are scarce, lipids become the predominant fuel source, providing long-lasting energy that keeps the body running. But, aside from providing energy, fats serve a variety of other purposes. They promote cell growth, protect the organs, and aid in food absorption. Essential fatty acids, which the body cannot make on its own, are essential for brain function, skin health, and even hormone production.

One might question how proteins and lipids fit into the carbohydrate-cycling problem. The beauty is in their adaptability. Proteins support muscle repair and growth on high-carb days, when the body is flooded with glucose, while fats, in moderation, give critical nutrients and keep the body content. Their roles become even more prominent on low-carb days. Proteins satisfy hunger, preventing the desire to grab for a quick carb fix, while fats take center stage, providing the majority of the body's energy.

It's a delicate balance that necessitates mindfulness and listening to the body's indications. For example, after an intense workout on a high-carb day, one may seek a protein-rich supper, indicating the body's need for muscle repair. A yearning for avocados or nuts on a low-carb day may signal the body's demand for sustained energy from fats.

It's critical to remember that this trip isn't simply about carbs as we negotiate the various pathways of carb-cycling. It's a comprehensive approach in which every nutrient is important, every meal is an opportunity to nourish the body, and mindfulness and attunement pave the way for optimal health. Proteins and lipids are co-stars in this nutrient dance, shining brilliantly and ensuring that the body remains vibrant, energized, and in sync with its nutritional needs.

Carb Timing: When and How Much to Eat

Timing is like to a maestro conducting an orchestra, ensuring each instrument plays its role at the precise moment, creating a perfect tune. Similarly, carbohydrate intake isn't just a matter of when you feel like it in the area of carb-cycling; it's a calculated decision aimed to optimize the body's metabolic responses and feed it for optimal performance.

Consider standing at the edge of a tranquil lake at morning. The only sound is the soft lapping of water against the shore. The world, and your body, awaken when the sun rises, producing a golden hue. This is the time when your body is calm but responsive, making it an ideal time to introduce carbohydrates, especially if you're planning a morning workout. Carbohydrates will not only fuel your exercise but will also jumpstart your metabolism for the day ahead.

However, the story does not finish there. The body's requirement for carbs ebbs and flows throughout the day, much like the natural rhythms. After a workout, the body is poised to absorb nutrients, particularly carbohydrates, to restore glycogen stores and aid muscle repair, which is known as the "anabolic window." It is a period when carbs are less likely to be stored as fat and more likely to be used for recovery and energy.

The metabolic rate slows down as evening approaches and the body prepares for rest. Consuming a lot of carbs during this time, especially if you're sedentary, might not be the best idea. Instead, focus on proteins and healthy fats, allowing your body to use these nutrients for repair and recuperation while you sleep.

But how much should you eat? There is no one-size-fits-all solution. It's a delicate balance that's influenced by things like individual metabolic rates, physical activity levels, and specific goals like weight loss, muscle building, or maintenance. Carbohydrate consumption may be higher for someone who engages in high-intensity training, whereas someone who has a sedentary lifestyle may benefit from a more controlled approach.

Carb timing in the context of carb-cycling is, in essence, an art, a dance of listening to one's body, knowing its rhythms, and feeding it with the proper fuel at the right moment. It's about being in tune with oneself, making informed decisions, and realizing that in the world of nutrition, timing is more than simply the ticking of the clock; it's the strategic symphony of nutrient intake.

Chapter 4: Overcoming Weight and Fitness Plateaus

No matter how well you prepare, there will always be obstacles on your fitness journey. One of the most difficult is reaching a plateau. At this juncture, determination is tested more severely than ever before, as the initial excitement fades in the face of prolonged inertia. Although scary, plateaus can be overcome. The theory and tactics behind breaking through these impasses are explored in depth in this chapter. Using carb cycling as our primary method, we'll discuss how to readjust our strategy for maintaining progress toward our health goals. This chapter provides insights, assistance, and inspiration to press through, from learning about the body's adaptive mechanisms to customizing carb-cycling to rekindle progress.

The Science of Weight Loss Plateaus

Every voyage, no matter how exciting, has periods of inactivity. Consider hiking in a large, lovely forest. Initially, each step you take takes you deeper into its splendor, with each turn providing a new, spectacular perspective. But then you find yourself traveling in circles, seeing the same trees and trails, and feeling as though you're not making any progress. This is the weight loss plateau - a moment in which, despite your best efforts, the scales don't budge and the mirror shows the same image day after day.

But why is this happening? Why does our body, which had before responded so brilliantly to our efforts, appear to abruptly hit the brakes? The solution is hidden deep inside our biology, sewn into the very fabric of evolution and survival.

Our body's intrinsic yearning for equilibrium lies at the center of it all. This is the body's system for maintaining internal stability in the face of external disturbances. When you start losing weight quickly, your body views it as a potential threat. In terms of evolution, our forefathers frequently encountered starvation. Rapid weight loss may indicate to the body that food is scarce, causing it to lower its metabolic rate in order to conserve energy. This is a survival strategy that ensures survival through difficult times.

Another factor is a drop in leptin, a hormone generated by fat cells. As you lose weight, your fat cells shrink, resulting in less leptin production. Leptin is essential for hunger and metabolic regulation. Lower leptin levels alert the brain to the fact that energy stores are depleted, resulting in increased appetite and lower energy expenditure.

Weight reduction plateaus can also be caused by muscle loss. When you lose weight, especially if you don't exercise, you're more likely to lose muscle mass as well as fat. Because muscles are metabolically active, meaning they burn calories even while resting, a loss of muscular mass might result in a slower metabolism.

As you lose weight, your body requires fewer calories to maintain your new weight. If you continue to consume the same number of calories that you did when you began your weight reduction journey, you will eventually reach a point where calorie intake equals calorie expenditure, resulting in a plateau.

But, beyond the science and biology, there is also the human factor to consider. It's natural to feel complacent as we advance through our weight reduction journey. Perhaps we begin to skip exercises, or perhaps we allow ourselves a few more indulgences, reasoning that a little here and there won't hurt. These minor adjustments can pile up over time and contribute to the plateau.

Understanding the science of weight loss plateaus is not about blaming or feeling disappointed. It is all about empowerment. It's about understanding that our bodies are complex, dynamic systems rather than machines that respond predictably to inputs. They have rhythms, cycles, and patterns that have evolved over millions of years.

So, if you're stuck in a weight loss rut, take a time to enjoy the beauty that is your body. Recognize that it is acting in your best interests. And, armed with an understanding of why plateaus occur, you can approach them as challenges to be understood, accepted, and eventually overcome.

How Carb-Cycling Acts as a Metabolic Reset

To understand the wonder of carb-cycling, we must first understand the complex dance of hormones, energy, and metabolism that occurs within us. Our bodies are constantly in motion, responding to the food we eat, the activities we engage in, and even the thoughts we have. Carbohydrates, as a key source of energy, play an important part in this dance. They have a significant impact on our metabolism and affect everything from our energy levels to our mood.

When we eat carbs, our bodies convert them into simpler sugars, typically glucose. This glucose enters our bloodstream, causing our pancreas to release insulin, a hormone that aids in glucose uptake by our cells. This procedure is smooth and efficient in a well-tuned metabolism. However, things can go wrong when the metabolism is out of sync. Excess carbohydrate consumption, particularly refined carbohydrate consumption, can cause insulin spikes and crashes, energy swings, and, over time, insulin resistance. This is the stage in which the body's reaction to insulin decreases, resulting in greater blood sugar levels and a slew of metabolic problems.

Here comes carb-cycling. Carb-cycling is fundamentally about altering carbohydrate consumption. Some days you eat more carbs, while others you eat less. This is not a random oscillation, but rather a planned alternation meant to maximize the benefits of both high and low carb days.

You fuel your body on high carb days by replacing glycogen stores in muscles, supporting strenuous exercises, and optimizing muscular growth. The carbohydrate surge also causes a transient boost in insulin, which, when timed correctly, can be anabolic, aiding in muscle repair and growth.

The magic intensifies on low carb days. When carbohydrate consumption is limited, the body turns to stored fat for energy. Insulin levels fall, allowing fat cells to release stored fat for fuel. Furthermore, low carb days might boost insulin sensitivity, ensuring that when you do ingest carbs, they are used more efficiently.

But wait, there's more. The cycle of high and low carb days causes a metabolic ebb and flow. It keeps the body guessing, preventing it from falling into a routine. This is important since our bodies are extremely adaptable. When faced with a constant stimulus, such as a fixed calorie intake or a consistent type of diet, our bodies react, resulting in plateaus. Carbohydrate cycling disrupts this predictability by acting as a metabolic reset.

This reset is both physiological and psychological. The diet's cyclical nature might be mentally rejuvenating. Instead of feeling deprived, as is frequent in many restrictive diets, folks anticipate a high carb day. This can improve diet adherence, making it more sustainable in the long run.

Carb-cycling can result in increased energy levels. Strategic carbohydrate consumption ensures that you have energy when you need it, such as on intensive workout days, while also allowing you to reap the benefits of fat metabolism on low carb days. This can result in sustained energy levels without the crashes that are commonly linked with heavy carb diets.

Carb-cycling is analogous to a symphony, with high and low carb days serving as contrasting notes in a harmonic metabolic melody. It honors the body's adaptable nature, works in harmony with our hormonal rhythms, and provides a long-term solution to weight management and metabolic health.

For those just starting out on this adventure, it's critical to approach carb-cycling with curiosity and patience. It's not just about counting carbs, but also about comprehending their significance, listening in to how different carb levels feel, and adjusting based on personal experiences and goals. We'll go deeper into the complexities of carb-cycling in the next chapters, providing insights, guidance, and recipes to make this journey both informative and tasty.

Tailoring Carb-Cycling to Break Through Stagnation

Starting a fitness journey is exciting. The early days, full with dedication and passion, frequently produce obvious results. The scale drops, muscles begin to define, and there is a renewed vigor that pervades daily activities. However, as many people can attest, there comes a point in this trip when progress appears to come to a halt. The scale refuses to budge, workouts become tedious, and the enthusiasm that once pushed the journey appears to have faded. This is the dreaded plateau, a stage in which results are elusive despite constant efforts.

Understanding plateaus necessitates a thorough examination of our bodies' adaptive systems. Our bodies are adaptability wonders. When exposed to a new stimulus, such as a diet modification or a new fitness routine, they respond, adjust, and evolve. However, as the stimulation becomes habitual, the body reaches its balance, and the previously observed rapid fluctuations begin to settle down.

Carb-cycling, with its cyclic oscillation between high and low carb days, provides a dynamic nutritional approach. But, like any other regimen, it is susceptible to the body's adaptive abilities. So, how does one adapt carb-cycling to break out of this rut?

The key is to recognize that carb-cycling is not a one-size-fits-all solution. It's a framework, a guideline that can and should be tweaked in response to individual reactions. It's critical for newcomers to understand that the body's response to carb-cycling will change over time. Carbohydrate ratios that previously produced results may need to be adjusted. The duration of the high and low carb stages may need to be adjusted. And the overall calorie intake, which is controlled by carbs, may need to be adjusted.

Introducing periodic carb refeeds is one effective method. A carb refeed, as opposed to the normal high carb day, comprises a purposeful, considerable increase in carb intake. This quick increase might stimulate the metabolism, resuming the fat-burning process and breaking the plateau. It's like throwing a curveball into the body's newly achieved homeostasis.

Another method is to change the duration of the low carb phase. Extending the low carb period by a day or two, followed by a brief high carb phase, can boost fat metabolism by forcing the body to use stored fat reserves for energy.

It's also worth mentioning that, while carbohydrates are the focus, other macronutrients play a role. Protein and fat intake should be adjusted on a regular basis, along with carbohydrate intake. Increased protein consumption, for example, during extended low carb phases helps preserve muscle mass, ensuring that the weight reduction is predominantly from fat.

Finally, it is critical to listen to one's body. Keeping track of energy levels, mood swings, and even sleep quality can provide insight into how the body is reacting to the present carb-cycling routine. These cues can be used to direct modifications, ensuring that the strategy remains effective and sustainable.

Breaking through a plateau involves a combination of science, intuition, and a dash of experimenting. It's about understanding that, while carb-cycling provides a solid foundation, it's the little, individual modifications that make it genuinely revolutionary.

Chapter 5: Mastering Meal Planning and Prep

Starting a carb-cycling adventure entails more than just learning the science of carbs and the benefits of cycling them. It's also a matter of practicality. How can you incorporate this dietary strategy into your daily life, especially when time is of the essence? Chapter 5 goes deeply into the problem, presenting concrete strategies to make carb-cycling not only doable but also fun. This chapter offers a complete guide to meal planning and preparation, covering everything from the art of menu planning to the complexities of ingredient swaps. Whether you're a seasoned chef or just getting started in the kitchen, the insights and suggestions presented here will help you handle the culinary side of carb-cycling with confidence and flair.

The Basics of Crafting a Carb-Cycling Menu

Setting off on a carb-cycling adventure is like to setting sail on unexplored waters. While scientifically sound and increasingly popular, the concept might be intimidating, especially for those just starting out in the wide ocean of dietary options. But don't worry, the essence of carb-cycling rests in its adjustability and freedom. It's not about imposing severe rules, but about finding your own rhythm and knowing your body's demands. The menu - the daily blueprint of your carb-cycling journey - is at the heart of this rhythm.

Creating a carb-cycling menu is an art as much as a science. cooking's an art because cooking necessitates imagination, a dash of culinary passion, and the skill to weave components together to create meals that satiate, nourish, and delight. It's a science since it necessitates knowledge of macronutrients, the role of carbohydrates in our physiology, and the capacity to customize intake to individual needs and goals.

So, where do you start?

Knowing Your Carbohydrate Threshold

It's critical to establish your carb threshold before digging into recipes and meal plans. This is the maximum amount of carbs you may eat while still meeting your goals, whether they are weight loss, muscle gain, or maintenance. For those looking to lose weight, the threshold may be lower on low-carb days and progressively increase on high-carb days to refuel and replace glycogen stores. Remember that these figures are not set in stone. They are a beginning point that can be adjusted based on progress and how one feels.

Carbohydrate Sources Should Be Diversified

Once you've established a rough estimate of your carb intake, the next step is to diversify your carb sources. Carbohydrates are not all made equal. While pastries and sugary cereals include carbohydrates, they lack the nutritional value of quinoa, sweet potatoes, or berries. Choose raw, unprocessed sources. These not only provide long-lasting energy but also necessary vitamins, minerals, and fiber.

Protein and fats must be balanced.

While carbohydrates are the focus, proteins and lipids play important supporting functions. Increased protein intake on low-carb days can help sustain muscle mass and keep you nourished. Fats, due to their increased caloric density, can offer the energy that the lowered carbs lack. Avocados, nuts, seeds, and fatty fish are all high in omega-3 fatty acids. While protein intake remains constant on high-carb days, lipids can be modestly lowered to meet the higher carb intake.

Paying Attention to Your Body's Cues

It's critical to pay attention to your body's cues while you plan your food. Some days, you may crave more carbs, while others, you may crave protein-rich foods. These cravings aren't random. They are your body's way of communicating with you about its needs. While sticking to the plan is vital, a little modification based on true physical indications can go a long way toward making the diet durable and effective.

Including Variation

Monotony is a common stumbling block in any diet. Eating the same meals every day might cause dietary weariness and even nutritional deficits. Aim for variety while preparing your carb-cycling menu. Rotate carb sources, explore with other cuisines, and don't be afraid to try new recipes. This not only keeps the diet interesting, but it also ensures a wider range of nutrients.

Preparation is essential.

Planning is one of the keys to successful carb-cycling. While spontaneity is the spice of life, a little planning can be a game changer when it comes to dietary tactics. Make time every week to plan your meals. This can include quantity cooking, prepping supplies, or simply sketching out a menu. When hunger strikes, this proactive strategy decreases the likelihood of opting for harmful, handy options.

Keeping Hydrated

While not directly related to menu planning, hydration is critical in carb-cycling. Because carbohydrates hold water, you may notice a little rise in weight on high-carb days. Staying hydrated allows your body to handle carbs more efficiently, promotes digestion, and even aids in muscle repair.

Creating a carb-cycling menu entails more than just counting carbs. It's about understanding their function, balancing them with other macronutrients, and preparing meals that you enjoy. It's about enjoying the road, appreciating each meal, and recognizing minor triumphs along the way. Carb-cycling may be transformed from a scary endeavor into a fascinating, fulfilling, and satisfying experience with a little information, planning, and a dash of culinary flair.

Ingredient Swaps and Kitchen Hacks

For many people, the kitchen is a haven. It's a place where inspiration meets nourishment, where the alchemy of cooking transforms simple materials into filling meals. However, for those starting out on a carb-cycling path, the kitchen can be a maze full with potential hazards and hurdles. How can one navigate this maze while ensuring that each meal meets the day's carb targets without sacrificing taste or nutrition? The solution is to learn the art of ingredient swapping and to embrace a few kitchen hacks.

The Substitution Effect

Substitution is about innovation, not deprivation. It's all about finding alternatives that not only match your carb-cycling aims, but also elevate your culinary creations. Let's look at some of these game changers:

Flour Substitutes: While traditional wheat flour is a kitchen staple in many households, it is heavy in carbohydrates. That doesn't mean you have to say goodbye to pancakes, muffins, and bread. Low-carb alternatives include almond flour, coconut flour, and flaxseed meal. Each provides a distinct flavor and texture to your recipes, providing depth and richness.

Rice Reimagined: Rice, a popular comfort dish, can be heavy in carbohydrates. But what if you could experience the texture and feel of rice without the added carbs? Here comes cauliflower rice. Cauliflower changes into a rice-like consistency when grated and sautéed, making it ideal for stir-fries, casseroles, and even sushi rolls.

Pasta Options: Don't worry, pasta connoisseurs. Low-carb alternatives to typical pasta include zoodles (zucchini noodles), spaghetti squash, and shirataki noodles. Each has its own texture and flavor profile, ensuring that your pasta recipes remain as varied and delicious as they always have been.

Kitchen Hacks That Work

Aside from item substitutions, a few kitchen tricks might make your carb-cycling trip easier and more enjoyable:

Batch Cooking: One of the most difficult aspects of carb-cycling is ensuring that each meal corresponds to the day's carb targets. Batch cooking can be a lifesaver in this situation. Preparing meals ahead of time not only saves time but also ensures that you always have a carb-appropriate meal on hand. This may include roasting some low-carb vegetables, grilling some meats, or making a pot of soup.

Herbs & spices: While carb-cycling necessitates careful control of macronutrient consumption, it does not necessitate bland meals. Herbs and spices are almost carb-free and may change even the most basic foods. These culinary friends ensure that your meals are always delectable, whether it's the warmth of cinnamon in a breakfast smoothie, the acidity of fresh basil in a salad, or the smokiness of paprika on grilled chicken.

Invest in Good Storage: When it comes to meal prep or preserving leftover ingredient swaps, good storage solutions are essential. To keep your food fresh, invest in airtight containers. This not only reduces food waste, but it also ensures that your meals remain as wonderful as when they were initially cooked.

Embrace the Digital Age: There are a plethora of applications and digital tools available to assist you in tracking your carb intake, finding recipes, and even offering item switch suggestions. While nothing beats the thrill of thumbing through a treasured cookbook, these digital aides can be invaluable, especially when you're just getting started with carb cycling.

Carbohydrate cycling, while an organized dietary approach, does not have to be rigid or restricted. It can be a wonderful culinary journey with the appropriate food swaps and kitchen techniques. It's about seeing each meal as an opportunity, a blank canvas where creativity, nutrition, and taste can all come together. And as you learn these substitutions and workarounds, you'll not only be better prepared to navigate the carb-cycling maze, but you'll also rediscover the joy of cooking in its simplest form - as an expression of love, caring, and nourishment.

Batch Cooking and Storage Tips for Busy Lives

Finding time to cook healthful meals on a regular basis can seem like a Herculean challenge in today's hectic world. Work, family, and personal commitments can leave us with little energy or desire to spend hours in the kitchen. Nonetheless, the desire to follow a carb-cycling diet and eat healthful, home-cooked meals remains strong. So, how can one balance these two diametrically opposed forces? The solution lies in batch cooking and clever storage.

Consider a world in which you can spend a few hours one day a week and have meals prepared for the next seven days. This is not a pipe dream; it is the reality of batch cooking. You may ensure that you always have a carb-appropriate meal on hand by making large amounts of food at once and storing it properly, even on the busiest of days.

The Science of Batch Cooking

Batch cooking entails more than simply preparing big quantities of food. It's a strategic approach that necessitates strategy, organization, and a little culinary imagination. Begin by creating a weekly menu. Consider the carb-cycling timetable and make sure your meals correspond to the high-carb and low-carb days. Make a detailed shopping list when you've decided on a menu. This not only saves time but also lowers the likelihood of making impulse purchases that are contrary to the diet.

When it comes to cooking, multitasking is essential. While a pot of soup simmers on one burner, roast some veggies and possibly grill some protein. The goal is to make the best use of kitchen appliances and time. Also, keep in mind that not everything needs to be totally cooked. Vegetables, for example, can be parboiled and then rapidly sautéed or roasted on the day you intend to eat them.

Keeping Things Safely

The success of batch cooking is dependent on proper storage. After all, the last thing you want is for the food to spoil after you've spent hours preparing it. Purchase high-quality airtight containers. These not only keep the food fresh, but they also keep cross-contamination at bay. Another critical issue is labeling. Mark each container clearly with the contents and the date of preparation. This ensures that you consume the meals while they are still fresh and also aids in meal planning based on the carb-cycling cycle.

Consider freezing for longer storage periods. Soups and casseroles, for example, freeze well. Remember to leave some space in the container because most foods expand when frozen. Simply thaw in the refrigerator and warm when ready to dine.

How to Make It Work for You

Batch cooking and wise storage are not hard and fast rules. They are adjustable and should be adapted to the needs of the individual. Start small if the thought of spending hours in the kitchen is intimidating. Perhaps plan meals for three days rather than a week. You'll find a rhythm that works best for you with time and practice.

Batch cooking and clever storage are really about making the kitchen work for you. They are tools that allow you to enjoy home-cooked, carb-friendly meals no matter how hectic your life becomes. It is about ensuring that, even in the midst of modern life, nourishment and health are prioritized.

Chapter 6: Recipe Compendium

Energizing High-Carb Breakfasts

Banana Berry Oatmeal

PREPARATION TIME	COOKING TIME	SERVING
Min. 5	Min. 10	1

INGREDIENTS	DIRECTIONS
<ul><li>1 cup rolled oats</li><li>2 cups water</li><li>1 medium banana, sliced</li><li>1/2 cup mixed berries (strawberries, blueberries, raspberries)</li><li>1 tablespoon honey or maple syrup</li><li>1 tablespoon chia seeds</li><li>1/2 teaspoon cinnamon</li></ul>	1. In a saucepan, bring the water to a boil. Add the oats and reduce the heat to low. Cook for about 10 minutes, stirring occasionally, until the oats are soft and have absorbed most of the water. 2. Stir in the sliced banana, mixed berries, honey or maple syrup, chia seeds, and cinnamon. Cook for another 2-3 minutes until the fruits are warm. 3. Transfer to a bowl and serve hot.

PER SERVING

Calories: 450kcal	Fat: 7g	Carbs: 90g	Protein: 12g

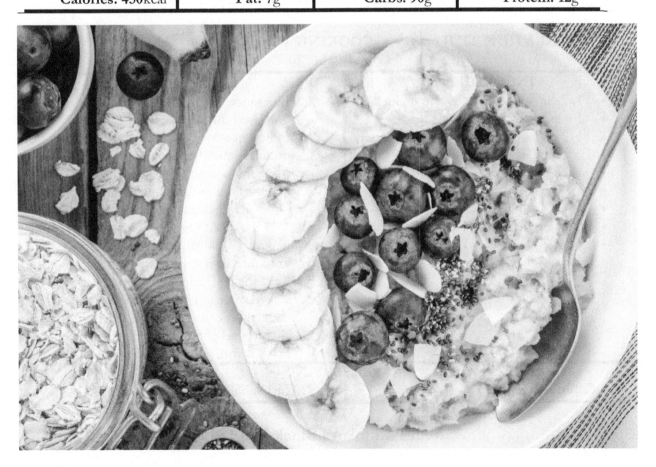

Whole Grain Pancakes with Apple and Nuts

PREPARATION TIME	COOKING TIME	SERVING
Min. 10	Min. 15	1

INGREDIENTS	DIRECTIONS
<ul><li>1 cup whole grain pancake mix</li><li>3/4 cup water</li><li>1 small apple, peeled and grated</li><li>2 tablespoons chopped nuts (almonds, walnuts, or pecans)</li><li>1 tablespoon vegetable oil</li><li>2 tablespoons maple syrup</li></ul>	1. In a bowl, combine the pancake mix, water, grated apple, and chopped nuts. Mix until just combined. Do not overmix. 2. Heat a non-stick skillet over medium heat and add a little vegetable oil. 3. Pour 1/4 cup of batter onto the skillet for each pancake. Cook until bubbles form on the surface, then flip and cook until golden brown on the other side. 4. Repeat with the remaining batter. 5. Serve the pancakes with maple syrup.

PER SERVING

Calories: 600kcal	Fat: 20g	Carbs: 100g	Protein: 15g

Quinoa and Vegetable Breakfast Bowl

PREPARATION TIME	COOKING TIME	SERVING
Min. 10	Min. 20	1

INGREDIENTS	DIRECTIONS
<ul><li>1/2 cup quinoa, rinsed and drained</li><li>1 cup water</li><li>1/2 cup diced vegetables (bell pepper, zucchini, cherry tomatoes)</li><li>1 tablespoon olive oil</li><li>1/4 teaspoon salt</li><li>1/4 teaspoon black pepper</li><li>2 tablespoons crumbled feta cheese</li><li>1 tablespoon chopped fresh parsley</li></ul>	1. In a saucepan, bring the water to a boil. Add the quinoa, reduce the heat to low, cover, and cook for about 15 minutes until the quinoa is cooked and the water is absorbed. 2. While the quinoa is cooking, heat the olive oil in a skillet over medium heat. Add the diced vegetables, salt, and pepper. Cook for about 5-7 minutes until the vegetables are tender. 3. Fluff the cooked quinoa with a fork and transfer to a bowl. Top with the cooked vegetables, crumbled feta cheese, and chopped parsley. 4. Serve warm.

PER SERVING

Calories: 450kcal	Fat: 20g	Carbs: 55g	Protein: 15g

Sweet Potato and Black Bean Hash

PREPARATION TIME	COOKING TIME	SERVING
Min. 10	Min. 20	1

INGREDIENTS

- 1 medium sweet potato, peeled and diced
- 1/2 cup canned black beans, drained and rinsed
- 1/2 small onion, diced
- 1 tablespoon olive oil
- 1/4 teaspoon paprika
- 1/4 teaspoon cumin
- Salt and pepper, to taste
- 2 tablespoons chopped fresh cilantro
- 1 tablespoon crumbled feta cheese

DIRECTIONS

1. In a large skillet, heat the olive oil over medium heat. Add the diced sweet potato and cook for about 10-12 minutes until tender, stirring occasionally.
2. Add the diced onion, paprika, cumin, salt, and pepper. Cook for another 5-7 minutes until the onion is soft and translucent.
3. Stir in the black beans and cook for another 2-3 minutes until heated through.
4. Transfer to a bowl and top with chopped cilantro and crumbled feta cheese.
5. Serve warm.

PER SERVING

Calories: 400kcal	Fat: 15g	Carbs: 60g	Protein: 12g

Spinach and Mushroom Omelette

PREPARATION TIME	COOKING TIME	SERVING
Min. 10	Min. 10	1

INGREDIENTS

- 2 large eggs
- 1/4 cup milk
- Salt and pepper, to taste
- 1 tablespoon butter
- 1/2 cup sliced mushrooms
- 1/2 cup fresh spinach, chopped
- 1/4 cup shredded cheddar cheese

DIRECTIONS

1. In a bowl, whisk together the eggs, milk, salt, and pepper.
2. In a non-stick skillet, melt the butter over medium heat. Add the sliced mushrooms and cook for about 5 minutes until tender.
3. Add the chopped spinach and cook for another 2-3 minutes until wilted.
4. Pour the egg mixture over the vegetables and cook for about 2-3 minutes until the edges start to set.
5. Sprinkle the shredded cheddar cheese over one half of the omelette. Fold the other half over the cheese.
6. Cook for another 2-3 minutes until the cheese is melted and the omelette is fully cooked.
7. Serve hot.

PER SERVING

Calories: 350kcal	Fat: 25g	Carbs: 10g	Protein: 20g

Peanut Butter and Banana Smoothie

PREPARATION TIME	COOKING TIME	SERVING
Min. 5	Min. 0	1

INGREDIENTS	DIRECTIONS
• 1 medium banana, sliced • 2 tablespoons peanut butter • 1 cup milk • 1 tablespoon honey or maple syrup • 1/2 teaspoon vanilla extract • 1 cup ice cubes	1. In a blender, combine the banana, peanut butter, milk, honey or maple syrup, vanilla extract, and ice cubes. 2. Blend until smooth and creamy. 3. Pour into a glass and serve immediately.

PER SERVING

Calories: 450kcal	Fat: 20g	Carbs: 60g	Protein: 15g

Apple and Cinnamon Porridge

PREPARATION TIME	COOKING TIME	SERVING
Min. 5	Min. 10	1

INGREDIENTS	DIRECTIONS
• 1/2 cup rolled oats • 1 cup milk • 1 small apple, peeled and grated • 1 tablespoon honey or maple syrup • 1/2 teaspoon cinnamon	1. In a saucepan, combine the oats, milk, grated apple, honey or maple syrup, and cinnamon. Bring to a boil, then reduce the heat to low and simmer for about 10 minutes until the oats are soft and the porridge is creamy.

- 1 tablespoon chopped nuts (almonds, walnuts, or pecans)

2. Transfer to a bowl and top with chopped nuts.
3. Serve hot.

PER SERVING			
Calories: 350kcal	Fat: 10g	Carbs: 60g	Protein: 10g

Berry and Yogurt Parfait

PREPARATION TIME Min. 10	COOKING TIME Min. 0	SERVING 1

INGREDIENTS	DIRECTIONS
• 1 cup mixed berries (strawberries, blueberries, raspberries) • 1 cup Greek yogurt • 2 tablespoons granola • 1 tablespoon honey or maple syrup	1. In a glass or jar, layer half of the Greek yogurt at the bottom. 2. Add a layer of half of the mixed berries, then a layer of half of the granola, and drizzle with half of the honey or maple syrup. 3. Repeat the layers with the remaining ingredients. 4. Serve immediately or refrigerate for later use.

PER SERVING			
Calories: 350kcal	Fat: 5g	Carbs: 60g	Protein: 20g

Avocado and Egg Toast

PREPARATION TIME Min. 5	COOKING TIME Min. 5	SERVING 1

INGREDIENTS	DIRECTIONS
• 1 slice whole grain bread • 1/2 avocado, mashed • 1 large egg • Salt and pepper, to taste • 1 tablespoon chopped fresh herbs (parsley, chives, or cilantro)	1. Toast the bread to your liking. 2. Spread the mashed avocado on the toast. 3. In a non-stick skillet, cook the egg to your liking (sunny side up, over easy, or scrambled). 4. Place the cooked egg on top of the avocado. 5. Season with salt and pepper and sprinkle with chopped herbs. 6. Serve immediately.

PER SERVING			
Calories: 300kcal	Fat: 20g	Carbs: 20g	Protein: 10g

Banana and Nut Muffins

PREPARATION TIME Min. 15	COOKING TIME Min. 20	SERVING 1

INGREDIENTS	DIRECTIONS
• 1 cup whole wheat flour • 1 teaspoon baking powder • 1/2 teaspoon baking soda • 1/4 teaspoon salt • 2 ripe bananas, mashed • 1/2 cup brown sugar • 1/4 cup melted butter • 1 large egg • 1/2 teaspoon vanilla extract • 1/2 cup chopped nuts (walnuts, pecans, or almonds)	1. Preheat the oven to 350°F (175°C) and line a muffin tin with paper liners. 2. In a bowl, combine the flour, baking powder, baking soda, and salt. 3. In another bowl, mix together the mashed bananas, brown sugar, melted butter, egg, and vanilla extract. 4. Add the wet ingredients to the dry ingredients and mix until just combined. Do not overmix. 5. Fold in the chopped nuts. 6. Divide the batter among the muffin cups. 7. Bake for 20-25 minutes until a toothpick inserted into the center of a muffin comes out clean. 8. Remove from the oven and let cool completely.

PER SERVING			
Calories: 250kcal	Fat: 10g	Carbs: 35g	Protein: 5g

Chocolate and Peanut Butter Smoothie

PREPARATION TIME	COOKING TIME	SERVING
Min. 5	Min. 0	1

INGREDIENTS	DIRECTIONS
• 1 medium banana, sliced • 2 tablespoons peanut butter • 1 cup milk • 1 tablespoon cocoa powder • 1 tablespoon honey or maple syrup • 1 cup ice cubes	1. In a blender, combine the banana, peanut butter, milk, cocoa powder, honey or maple syrup, and ice cubes. 2. Blend until smooth and creamy. 3. Pour into a glass and serve immediately.

PER SERVING			
Calories: 450kcal	Fat: 20g	Carbs: 60g	Protein: 15g

Apple and Cinnamon Oatmeal

PREPARATION TIME	COOKING TIME	SERVING
Min. 5	Min. 10	1

INGREDIENTS	DIRECTIONS
• 1/2 cup rolled oats • 1 cup milk or water • 1 apple, peeled and chopped • 1 tablespoon brown sugar • 1/2 teaspoon cinnamon • 1/4 teaspoon nutmeg	1. In a saucepan, combine the oats, milk or water, chopped apple, brown sugar, cinnamon, and nutmeg. 2. Bring to a boil, then reduce the heat to low and simmer for 5-7 minutes until the oats are tender and the liquid is absorbed.

- 1 tablespoon chopped nuts (almonds, walnuts, or pecans

3. Stir in the chopped nuts.
4. Serve hot.

PER SERVING			
Calories: 350kcal	Fat: 10g	Carbs: 60g	Protein: 10g

Berry and Nut Smoothie

PREPARATION TIME	COOKING TIME	SERVING
Min. 5	Min. 0	1

INGREDIENTS	DIRECTIONS
• 1 cup mixed berries (strawberries, blueberries, raspberries) • 1 cup milk or yogurt • 1 tablespoon honey or maple syrup • 1/4 cup chopped nuts (almonds, walnuts, or pecans) • 1 cup ice cubes	1. In a blender, combine the mixed berries, milk or yogurt, honey or maple syrup, chopped nuts, and ice cubes. 2. Blend until smooth and creamy. 3. Pour into a glass and serve immediately.

PER SERVING			
Calories: 350kcal	Fat: 15g	Carbs: 50g	Protein: 10g

Peanut Butter and Banana Pancakes

PREPARATION TIME	COOKING TIME	SERVING
Min. 10	Min. 10	1

INGREDIENTS	DIRECTIONS
• 1 cup all-purpose flour • 1 tablespoon sugar • 1 teaspoon baking powder • 1/2 teaspoon baking soda • 1/4 teaspoon salt • 1 cup milk • 1 large egg • 2 tablespoons melted butter • 1/2 cup mashed banana • 2 tablespoons peanut butter • 1/2 teaspoon vanilla extract	1. In a bowl, combine the flour, sugar, baking powder, baking soda, and salt. 2. In another bowl, mix together the milk, egg, melted butter, mashed banana, peanut butter, and vanilla extract. 3. Add the wet ingredients to the dry ingredients and mix until just combined. Do not overmix. 4. Heat a non-stick skillet over medium heat and lightly grease with butter or oil. 5. Pour 1/4 cup of batter onto the skillet and cook until bubbles form on the surface, then flip and cook until golden brown. 6. Repeat with the remaining batter. 7. Serve hot with your favorite toppings.

PER SERVING			
Calories: 350kcal	Fat: 15g	Carbs: 45g	Protein: 10g

Mango and Coconut Smoothie

PREPARATION TIME Min. 5	COOKING TIME Min. 0	SERVING 1

INGREDIENTS	DIRECTIONS
• 1 cup chopped mango • 1/2 cup coconut milk • 1/2 cup yogurt • 1 tablespoon honey or maple syrup • 1 cup ice cubes	1. In a blender, combine the mango, coconut milk, yogurt, honey or maple syrup, and ice cubes. 2. Blend until smooth and creamy. 3. Pour into a glass and serve immediately.

PER SERVING			
Calories: 350kcal	Fat: 15g	Carbs: 50g	Protein:5 g

Avocado and Tomato Salad

PREPARATION TIME Min. 10	COOKING TIME Min. 0	SERVING 1

INGREDIENTS	DIRECTIONS
• 1 avocado, peeled and sliced • 1 tomato, sliced • 1/4 cup fresh basil, chopped • 2 tablespoons olive oil • 1 tablespoon balsamic vinegar • Salt and pepper, to taste	1. In a bowl, combine the avocado, tomato, and fresh basil. 2. Drizzle the olive oil and balsamic vinegar on top. 3. Season with salt and pepper. 4. Serve immediately.

PER SERVING			
Calories: 350kcal	Fat: 30g	Carbs: 15g	Protein: 5g

Protein-Packed Low-Carb Breakfasts

Scrambled Eggs with Spinach and Feta

PREPARATION TIME Min. 5	COOKING TIME Min.10	SERVING 1

INGREDIENTS	DIRECTIONS
• 3 large eggs • 1 cup fresh spinach, chopped • 1/4 cup feta cheese, crumbled • 1 tablespoon olive oil • Salt and pepper, to taste	1. In a bowl, whisk the eggs and season with salt and pepper. 2. Heat the olive oil in a non-stick skillet over medium heat. 3. Add the spinach and cook for 2-3 minutes until wilted. 4. Add the eggs and cook until scrambled. 5. Sprinkle the feta cheese on top. 6. Serve hot.

PER SERVING

Calories: 350kcal	Fat: 25g	Carbs: 5g	Protein: 25g

Avocado and Smoked Salmon Roll-Ups

PREPARATION TIME Min. 10	COOKING TIME Min. 0	SERVING 1

INGREDIENTS	DIRECTIONS
• 1 avocado, peeled and sliced • 3 slices smoked salmon • 1 tablespoon cream cheese • 1 tablespoon chopped fresh dill • Salt and pepper, to taste	1. Lay the smoked salmon slices on a flat surface. 2. Spread the cream cheese on each slice. 3. Arrange the avocado slices on top. 4. Season with salt and pepper. 5. Sprinkle the fresh dill on top. 6. Roll the smoked salmon slices tightly and secure with a toothpick. 7. Serve immediately.

PER SERVING

Calories: 350kcal	Fat: 30g	Carbs: 10g	Protein: 15g

Almond and Coconut Pancakes

PREPARATION TIME Min. 10	COOKING TIME Min. 10	SERVING 1

INGREDIENTS	DIRECTIONS
• 1/2 cup almond flour • 1/4 cup shredded coconut • 2 large eggs • 1/4 cup almond milk • 1 tablespoon melted coconut oil • 1 teaspoon vanilla extract • 1/2 teaspoon baking powder • 1 tablespoon erythritol or other low-carb sweetener • Pinch of salt • Butter or coconut oil, for frying	1. In a bowl, combine the almond flour, shredded coconut, eggs, almond milk, melted coconut oil, vanilla extract, baking powder, erythritol, and salt. 2. Mix well until a smooth batter forms. 3. Heat a non-stick skillet over medium heat and add a little butter or coconut oil. 4. Pour a small amount of batter into the skillet and cook for 2-3 minutes on each side until golden brown. 5. Repeat with the remaining batter. 6. Serve hot with your favorite low-carb toppings.

PER SERVING

Calories: 350kcal	Fat: 30g	Carbs: 10g	Protein: 15g

Greek Yogurt and Berry Parfait

PREPARATION TIME Min. 5	COOKING TIME Min. 0	SERVING 1

INGREDIENTS	DIRECTIONS
• 1 cup Greek yogurt, unsweetened	

- 1/2 cup mixed berries (strawberries, blueberries, raspberries)
- 1 tablespoon chopped nuts (almonds, walnuts, or pecans)
- 1 tablespoon chia seeds
- 1 tablespoon erythritol or other low-carb sweetener

1. In a glass or jar, layer the Greek yogurt, mixed berries, chopped nuts, chia seeds, and erythritol.
2. Repeat the layers until the glass or jar is full.
3. Serve immediately or refrigerate for later use.

PER SERVING			
Calories: 350kcal	Fat: 15g	Carbs: 15g	Protein: 25g

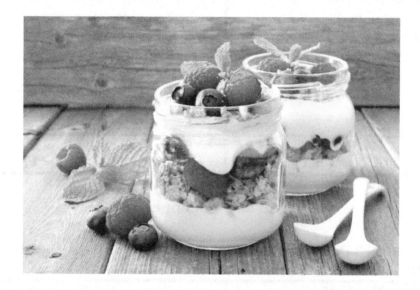

Egg and Sausage Breakfast Muffins

PREPARATION TIME	COOKING TIME	SERVING
Min. 10	Min. 20	1

INGREDIENTS	DIRECTIONS
<ul><li>6 large eggs</li><li>1/2 cup cooked sausage, crumbled</li><li>1/4 cup shredded cheese (cheddar, mozzarella, or feta)</li><li>1/4 cup chopped vegetables (bell peppers, zucchini, or spinach)</li><li>1/4 teaspoon salt</li><li>1/4 teaspoon pepper</li><li>Butter or coconut oil, for greasing</li></ul>	1. Preheat the oven to 350°F (175°C) and grease a muffin tin with butter or coconut oil. 2. In a bowl, whisk the eggs and season with salt and pepper. 3. Add the cooked sausage, shredded cheese, and chopped vegetables and mix well. 4. Divide the mixture evenly among the muffin cups. 5. Bake for 20-25 minutes until the eggs are fully cooked and the tops are golden brown. 6. Let cool for a few minutes before removing from the muffin tin. 7. Serve hot or refrigerate for later use.

PER SERVING			
Calories: 150kcal	Fat: 10g	Carbs: 2g	Protein: 10g

Smoked Salmon and Cream Cheese Omelette

PREPARATION TIME	COOKING TIME	SERVING
Min. 5	Min. 10	1

INGREDIENTS	DIRECTIONS
• 3 large eggs • 3 slices smoked salmon • 2 tablespoons cream cheese • 1 tablespoon chopped fresh chives • 1 tablespoon butter or coconut oil • Salt and pepper, to taste	1. In a bowl, whisk the eggs and season with salt and pepper. 2. Heat the butter or coconut oil in a non-stick skillet over medium heat. 3. Pour the eggs into the skillet and cook until the edges start to set. 4. Arrange the smoked salmon and cream cheese on one half of the omelette. 5. Sprinkle the fresh chives on top. 6. Fold the omelette in half and cook for another 2-3 minutes until fully cooked. 7. Serve hot.

PER SERVING			
Calories: 350kcal	Fat: 25g	Carbs: 5g	Protein: 25g

Almond and Berry Smoothie

PREPARATION TIME	COOKING TIME	SERVING
Min. 5	Min. 0	1

INGREDIENTS	DIRECTIONS
• 1 cup mixed berries (strawberries, blueberries, raspberries) • 1 cup almond milk, unsweetened • 1/4 cup almond butter • 1 tablespoon chia seeds • 1 tablespoon erythritol or other low-carb sweetener • 1 cup ice cubes	1. In a blender, combine the mixed berries, almond milk, almond butter, chia seeds, erythritol, and ice cubes. 2. Blend until smooth and creamy. 3. Pour into a glass and serve immediately.

PER SERVING			
Calories: 350kcal	Fat: 25g	Carbs: 15g	Protein: 20g

Chicken and Vegetable Stir-Fry

PREPARATION TIME	COOKING TIME	SERVING
Min. 10	Min. 10	1

INGREDIENTS	DIRECTIONS
• 1 chicken breast, sliced • 1 cup mixed vegetables (bell peppers, zucchini, broccoli) • 2 tablespoons soy sauce • 1 tablespoon olive oil • 1 teaspoon sesame seeds • Salt and pepper, to taste	1. Heat the olive oil in a non-stick skillet over medium heat. 2. Add the chicken slices and cook for 5-7 minutes until fully cooked. 3. Add the mixed vegetables and cook for another 3-5 minutes until tender. 4. Add the soy sauce and mix well. 5. Season with salt and pepper. 6. Sprinkle the sesame seeds on top. 7. Serve hot.

PER SERVING			
Calories: 350kcal	Fat: 15g	Carbs: 15g	Protein: 35g

Turkey and Cheese Roll-Ups

PREPARATION TIME Min. 5	COOKING TIME Min. 0	SERVING 1

INGREDIENTS	DIRECTIONS
• 3 slices turkey breast • 3 slices cheese (cheddar, mozzarella, or swiss) • 1/4 cup fresh spinach, chopped • 1 tablespoon mayonnaise • 1 tablespoon mustard • Salt and pepper, to taste	1. Lay the turkey slices on a flat surface. 2. Spread the mayonnaise and mustard on each slice. 3. Arrange the cheese and spinach on top. 4. Season with salt and pepper. 5. Roll the turkey slices tightly and secure with a toothpick. 6. Serve immediately.

PER SERVING			
Calories: 350kcal	Fat: 25g	Carbs: 5g	Protein: 25g

Egg and Sausage Breakfast Burrito

PREPARATION TIME Min. 10	COOKING TIME Min. 10	SERVING 1

INGREDIENTS	DIRECTIONS
• 1 low-carb tortilla • 2 large eggs • 1/4 cup cooked sausage, crumbled • 1/4 cup shredded cheese (cheddar, mozzarella, or feta) • 1/4 cup salsa • 1 tablespoon olive oil • Salt and pepper, to taste	1. In a bowl, whisk the eggs and season with salt and pepper. 2. Heat the olive oil in a non-stick skillet over medium heat. 3. Add the eggs and cook until scrambled. 4. Warm the tortilla in the skillet for 1-2 minutes on each side. 5. Arrange the scrambled eggs, sausage, cheese, and salsa on the tortilla. 6. Roll the tortilla tightly and secure with a toothpick.

7. Serve hot.

PER SERVING			
Calories: 350kcal	Fat: 25g	Carbs: 15g	Protein: 20g

Almond and Coconut Granola

PREPARATION TIME Min. 10	COOKING TIME Min. 20	SERVING 1

INGREDIENTS	DIRECTIONS
<ul><li>1 cup almonds, chopped</li><li>1/2 cup shredded coconut, unsweetened</li><li>1/4 cup pumpkin seeds</li><li>1/4 cup sunflower seeds</li><li>1/4 cup flaxseeds</li><li>1/4 cup melted coconut oil</li><li>1/4 cup erythritol or other low-carb sweetener</li><li>1 teaspoon cinnamon</li><li>1/2 teaspoon vanilla extract</li><li>Pinch of salt</li></ul>	1. Preheat the oven to 350°F (175°C) and line a baking tray with parchment paper. 2. In a bowl, combine the almonds, shredded coconut, pumpkin seeds, sunflower seeds, flaxseeds, melted coconut oil, erythritol, cinnamon, vanilla extract, and salt. 3. Mix well until all the ingredients are well coated. 4. Spread the mixture evenly on the baking tray. 5. Bake for 20-25 minutes until golden brown. 6. Let cool completely before breaking into clusters. 7. Store in an airtight container.

PER SERVING			
Calories: 200kcal	Fat: 15g	Carbs: 10g	Protein: 5g

Bacon and Egg Breakfast Cups

PREPARATION TIME Min. 10	COOKING TIME Min. 20	SERVING 1

INGREDIENTS	DIRECTIONS
<ul><li>6 slices bacon</li><li>6 large eggs</li><li>1/4 cup shredded cheese (cheddar, mozzarella, or feta)</li><li>1/4 cup chopped vegetables (bell peppers, zucchini, or spinach)</li><li>1/4 teaspoon salt</li><li>1/4 teaspoon pepper</li><li>Butter or coconut oil, for greasing</li></ul>	1. Preheat the oven to 350°F (175°C) and grease a muffin tin with butter or coconut oil. 2. Cook the bacon slices in a non-stick skillet over medium heat until partially cooked but still flexible. 3. Arrange the bacon slices in the muffin cups. 4. In a bowl, whisk the eggs and season with salt and pepper. 5. Add the shredded cheese and chopped vegetables and mix well. 6. Divide the mixture evenly among the muffin cups.

7. Bake for 20-25 minutes until the eggs are fully cooked and the tops are golden brown.
8. Let cool for a few minutes before removing from the muffin tin.
9. Serve hot or refrigerate for later use.

PER SERVING			
Calories: 150kcal	Fat: 10g	Carbs: 2g	Protein: 10g

Spinach and Feta Omelette

PREPARATION TIME Min. 5	COOKING TIME Min. 10	SERVING 1

INGREDIENTS	DIRECTIONS
• 3 large eggs • 1 cup fresh spinach, chopped • 1/4 cup feta cheese, crumbled • 1 tablespoon olive oil • Salt and pepper, to taste	1. In a bowl, whisk the eggs and season with salt and pepper. 2. Heat the olive oil in a non-stick skillet over medium heat. 3. Add the spinach and cook for 2-3 minutes until wilted. 4. Add the eggs and cook until the edges start to set. 5. Sprinkle the feta cheese on top. 6. Fold the omelette in half and cook for another 2-3 minutes until fully cooked. 7. Serve hot.

PER SERVING			
Calories: 350kcal	Fat: 25g	Carbs: 5g	Protein: 25g

Turkey and Avocado Wrap

PREPARATION TIME Min. 5	COOKING TIME Min. 0	SERVING 1

INGREDIENTS	DIRECTIONS
• 1 low-carb tortilla • 3 slices turkey breast • 1/2 avocado, peeled and sliced • 1/4 cup fresh spinach, chopped • 1 tablespoon mayonnaise • 1 tablespoon mustard • Salt and pepper, to taste Procedure:	1. Lay the tortilla on a flat surface. 2. Spread the mayonnaise and mustard on the tortilla. 3. Arrange the turkey slices, avocado, and spinach on top. 4. Season with salt and pepper. 5. Roll the tortilla tightly and secure with a toothpick. 6. Serve immediately.

PER SERVING			
Calories: 350kcal	Fat: 25g	Carbs: 15g	Protein: 20g

Vibrant High-Carb Lunches

Chickpea and Vegetable Stir-Fry

PREPARATION TIME	COOKING TIME	SERVING
Min. 10	Min. 15	1

INGREDIENTS	DIRECTIONS
• 1 cup chickpeas, cooked • 1 cup broccoli florets • 1/2 cup bell peppers, sliced • 1/2 cup carrots, sliced • 2 tbsp soy sauce • 1 tbsp olive oil • 1 tsp ginger, minced • 1 tsp garlic, minced • Salt and pepper to taste	1. Heat olive oil in a pan over medium heat. Add ginger and garlic and sauté for 1-2 minutes until fragrant. 2. Add broccoli, bell peppers, and carrots to the pan. Stir-fry for about 5-7 minutes until the vegetables are tender. 3. Add chickpeas, soy sauce, salt, and pepper. Stir well and cook for another 3-5 minutes. 4. Serve hot.

PER SERVING			
Calories: 400kcal	Fat: 12g	Carbs: 60g	Protein: 18g

Quinoa and Black Bean Salad

PREPARATION TIME	COOKING TIME	SERVING
Min. 10	Min. 20	1

INGREDIENTS	DIRECTIONS
• 1/2 cup quinoa, uncooked • 1 cup black beans, cooked • 1 cup cherry tomatoes, halved • 1/2 cup corn kernels • 1/4 cup red onion, chopped • 2 tbsp olive oil • 1 tbsp lemon juice • Salt and pepper to taste • 2 tbsp fresh cilantro, chopped	1. Cook quinoa according to package instructions. Set aside to cool. 2. In a large bowl, combine black beans, cherry tomatoes, corn, and red onion. 3. In a small bowl, whisk together olive oil, lemon juice, salt, and pepper. 4. Add quinoa and dressing to the vegetable mixture. Toss well to combine. 5. Garnish with fresh cilantro before serving.

PER SERVING			
Calories: 550kcal	Fat: 18g	Carbs: 80g	Protein: 20g

Sweet Potato and Lentil Curry

PREPARATION TIME	COOKING TIME	SERVING
Min. 10	Min. 30	1

INGREDIENTS

- 1 cup sweet potato, diced
- 1/2 cup lentils, uncooked
- 1 cup coconut milk
- 1 cup vegetable broth
- 1 tbsp curry powder
- 1 tsp turmeric
- 1 tbsp olive oil
- Salt and pepper to taste
- 2 tbsp fresh cilantro, chopped

DIRECTIONS

1. Heat olive oil in a pot over medium heat. Add sweet potato and cook for about 5 minutes until slightly softened.
2. Add lentils, coconut milk, vegetable broth, curry powder, turmeric, salt, and pepper. Bring to a boil, then reduce heat to low and simmer for about 20-25 minutes until the lentils and sweet potato are tender.
3. Garnish with fresh cilantro before serving.

PER SERVING

Calories: 600kcal	Fat: 25g	Carbs: 80g	Protein: 20g

Brown Rice and Vegetable Bowl

PREPARATION TIME	COOKING TIME	SERVING
Min. 10	Min. 20	1

INGREDIENTS

- 1/2 cup brown rice, uncooked
- 1 cup broccoli florets
- 1/2 cup bell peppers, sliced
- 1/2 cup snap peas
- 1/4 cup green onions, chopped
- 2 tbsp soy sauce
- 1 tbsp sesame oil
- 1 tbsp sesame seeds
- Salt and pepper to taste

DIRECTIONS

1. Cook brown rice according to package instructions. Set aside.
2. In a pan, heat sesame oil over medium heat. Add broccoli, bell peppers, and snap peas. Stir-fry for about 5-7 minutes until the vegetables are tender.
3. Add cooked rice, soy sauce, salt, and pepper. Stir well to combine.
4. Garnish with green onions and sesame seeds before serving.

PER SERVING

Calories: 500kcal	Fat: 15g	Carbs: 80g	Protein: 15g

Pasta Primavera

PREPARATION TIME	COOKING TIME	SERVING
Min. 10	Min. 20	1

INGREDIENTS

- 1 cup whole wheat pasta, uncooked
- 1/2 cup cherry tomatoes, halved
- 1/2 cup zucchini, sliced
- 1/2 cup bell peppers, sliced
- 1/4 cup red onion, chopped
- 2 tbsp olive oil
- 2 tbsp parmesan cheese, grated
- Salt and pepper to taste
- 2 tbsp fresh basil, chopped

DIRECTIONS

1. Cook pasta according to package instructions. Drain and set aside.
2. In a pan, heat olive oil over medium heat. Add cherry tomatoes, zucchini, bell peppers, and red onion. Cook for about 5-7 minutes until the vegetables are tender.
3. Add cooked pasta, parmesan cheese, salt, and pepper. Stir well to combine.

4. Garnish with fresh basil before serving.

PER SERVING			
Calories: 550kcal	Fat: 20g	Carbs: 80g	Protein: 20g

Vegetable and Bean Burrito

PREPARATION TIME Min. 10	COOKING TIME Min. 15	SERVING 1

INGREDIENTS	DIRECTIONS
• 1 whole wheat tortilla • 1/2 cup black beans, cooked • 1/2 cup corn kernels • 1/2 cup bell peppers, sliced • 1/4 cup red onion, chopped • 1/4 cup cheddar cheese, shredded • 2 tbsp salsa • 1 tbsp olive oil • Salt and pepper to taste	1. In a pan, heat olive oil over medium heat. Add bell peppers and red onion. Cook for about 5-7 minutes until the vegetables are tender. 2. Add black beans, corn, salt, and pepper. Stir well to combine. 3. Warm the tortilla in a dry pan over medium heat for about 1 minute on each side. 4. Spread salsa over the tortilla. Add the vegetable and bean mixture, and sprinkle with cheddar cheese. 5. Roll up the tortilla, folding in the sides as you go. 6. Serve warm.

PER SERVING			
Calories: 550kcal	Fat: 20g	Carbs: 80g	Protein: 20g

Lentil and Vegetable Stew

PREPARATION TIME Min. 10	COOKING TIME Min. 30	SERVING 1

INGREDIENTS	DIRECTIONS
• 1/2 cup lentils, uncooked • 1 cup vegetable broth • 1/2 cup carrots, sliced • 1/2 cup zucchini, sliced • 1/2 cup tomatoes, chopped • 1/4 cup red onion, chopped • 1 tbsp olive oil • 1 tsp cumin • Salt and pepper to taste • 2 tbsp fresh parsley, chopped	1. Heat olive oil in a pot over medium heat. Add red onion and cook for about 3-5 minutes until softened. 2. Add carrots, zucchini, tomatoes, lentils, vegetable broth, cumin, salt, and pepper. Bring to a boil, then reduce heat to low and simmer for about 20-25 minutes until the lentils and vegetables are tender. 3. Garnish with fresh parsley before serving.

PER SERVING			
Calories: 400kcal	Fat: 10g	Carbs: 60g	Protein: 20g

Vegetable and Quinoa Stir-Fry

PREPARATION TIME	COOKING TIME	SERVING
Min. 10	Min. 20	1

INGREDIENTS	DIRECTIONS
• 1/2 cup quinoa, uncooked • 1 cup broccoli florets • 1/2 cup bell peppers, sliced • 1/2 cup snap peas • 1/4 cup green onions, chopped • 2 tbsp soy sauce • 1 tbsp sesame oil • 1 tbsp sesame seeds • Salt and pepper to taste	1. Cook quinoa according to package instructions. Set aside. 2. In a pan, heat sesame oil over medium heat. Add broccoli, bell peppers, and snap peas. Stir-fry for about 5-7 minutes until the vegetables are tender. 3. Add cooked quinoa, soy sauce, salt, and pepper. Stir well to combine. 4. Garnish with green onions and sesame seeds before serving.

PER SERVING			
Calories: 500kcal	Fat: 15g	Carbs: 70g	Protein: 20g

Chickpea and Vegetable Curry

PREPARATION TIME	COOKING TIME	SERVING
Min. 10	Min. 20	1

INGREDIENTS	DIRECTIONS
• 1 cup chickpeas, cooked • 1 cup coconut milk • 1/2 cup bell peppers, sliced • 1/2 cup zucchini, sliced • 1/4 cup red onion, chopped • 2 tbsp curry paste • 1 tbsp olive oil • Salt and pepper to taste • 2 tbsp fresh cilantro, chopped	1. Heat olive oil in a pan over medium heat. Add red onion and cook for about 3-5 minutes until softened. 2. Add bell peppers and zucchini. Cook for about 5-7 minutes until the vegetables are tender. 3. Add chickpeas, coconut milk, curry paste, salt, and pepper. Stir well to combine and cook for another 5-7 minutes until heated through. 4. Garnish with fresh cilantro before serving.

PER SERVING			
Calories: 600kcal	Fat: 25g	Carbs: 80g	Protein: 20g

Pasta with Tomato and Basil Sauce

PREPARATION TIME	COOKING TIME	SERVING
Min. 10	Min. 20	1

INGREDIENTS

- 1 cup whole wheat pasta, uncooked
- 1 cup cherry tomatoes, halved
- 1/4 cup red onion, chopped
- 2 tbsp olive oil
- 2 tbsp parmesan cheese, grated
- Salt and pepper to taste
- 2 tbsp fresh basil, chopped

DIRECTIONS

1. Cook pasta according to package instructions. Drain and set aside.
2. In a pan, heat olive oil over medium heat. Add red onion and cook for about 3-5 minutes until softened.
3. Add cherry tomatoes, salt, and pepper. Cook for about 5-7 minutes until the tomatoes are softened.
4. Add cooked pasta, parmesan cheese, and fresh basil. Stir well to combine.
5. Serve warm.

PER SERVING

Calories: 550kcal	Fat: 20g	Carbs: 80g	Protein: 20g

Brown Rice and Bean Bowl

PREPARATION TIME	COOKING TIME	SERVING
Min. 10	Min. 20	1

INGREDIENTS

- 1/2 cup brown rice, uncooked
- 1 cup black beans, cooked
- 1/2 cup corn kernels
- 1/2 cup cherry tomatoes, halved
- 1/4 cup red onion, chopped
- 2 tbsp olive oil
- 1 tbsp lemon juice
- Salt and pepper to taste
- 2 tbsp fresh cilantro, chopped

DIRECTIONS

1. Cook brown rice according to package instructions. Set aside.
2. In a large bowl, combine black beans, corn, cherry tomatoes, and red onion.
3. In a small bowl, whisk together olive oil, lemon juice, salt, and pepper.
4. Add cooked rice and dressing to the vegetable mixture. Toss well to combine.
5. Garnish with fresh cilantro before serving.

PER SERVING

Calories: 550kcal	Fat: 18g	Carbs: 80g	Protein: 20g

Vegetable and Lentil Soup

PREPARATION TIME	COOKING TIME	SERVING
Min. 10	Min. 30	1

INGREDIENTS

- 1/2 cup lentils, uncooked
- 1 cup vegetable broth
- 1/2 cup carrots, sliced
- 1/2 cup zucchini, sliced
- 1/2 cup tomatoes, chopped
- 1/4 cup red onion, chopped
- 1 tbsp olive oil
- 1 tsp cumin
- Salt and pepper to taste

DIRECTIONS

1. Heat olive oil in a pot over medium heat. Add red onion and cook for about 3-5 minutes until softened.
2. Add carrots, zucchini, tomatoes, lentils, vegetable broth, cumin, salt, and pepper. Bring to a boil, then reduce heat to low and simmer for about 20-25 minutes until the lentils and vegetables are tender.

	• 2 tbsp fresh parsley, chopped	3. Garnish with fresh parsley before serving.

PER SERVING			
Calories: 400kcal	Fat: 10g	Carbs: 60g	Protein: 20g

Quinoa and Vegetable Salad

PREPARATION TIME Min. 10	COOKING TIME Min. 10	SERVING 1
INGREDIENTS	**DIRECTIONS**	
• 1/2 cup quinoa, uncooked • 1 cup cherry tomatoes, halved • 1/2 cup cucumber, sliced • 1/2 cup bell peppers, sliced • 1/4 cup red onion, chopped • 2 tbsp olive oil • 1 tbsp lemon juice • Salt and pepper to taste • 2 tbsp fresh parsley, chopped	1. Cook quinoa according to package instructions. Set aside to cool. 2. In a large bowl, combine cherry tomatoes, cucumber, bell peppers, and red onion. 3. In a small bowl, whisk together olive oil, lemon juice, salt, and pepper. 4. Add quinoa and dressing to the vegetable mixture. Toss well to combine. 5. Garnish with fresh parsley before serving.	

PER SERVING			
Calories: 500kcal	Fat: 18g	Carbs: 70g	Protein: 20g

Chickpea and Tomato Stew

PREPARATION TIME Min. 10	COOKING TIME Min. 20	SERVING 1
INGREDIENTS	**DIRECTIONS**	
• 1 cup chickpeas, cooked • 1 cup tomatoes, chopped • 1/2 cup bell peppers, sliced • 1/4 cup red onion, chopped • 1 cup vegetable broth • 1 tbsp olive oil • 1 tsp paprika • Salt and pepper to taste • 2 tbsp fresh cilantro, chopped	1. Heat olive oil in a pot over medium heat. Add red onion and cook for about 3-5 minutes until softened. 2. Add bell peppers, tomatoes, chickpeas, vegetable broth, paprika, salt, and pepper. Bring to a boil, then reduce heat to low and simmer for about 15-20 minutes until the vegetables are tender. 3. Garnish with fresh cilantro before serving.	

PER SERVING			
Calories: 400kcal	Fat: 12g	Carbs: 60g	Protein: 18g

Grilled Chicken Salad

PREPARATION TIME Min. 10	COOKING TIME Min. 15	SERVING 1

INGREDIENTS	DIRECTIONS
• 1 chicken breast • 2 cups mixed salad greens • 1/2 cup cherry tomatoes, halved • 1/4 cup cucumber, sliced • 1/4 cup red bell pepper, sliced • 1 tablespoon olive oil • 2 tablespoons balsamic vinegar • Salt and pepper to taste	1. Season the chicken breast with salt and pepper. Grill the chicken breast for about 6-7 minutes on each side or until fully cooked. Slice the chicken into strips. 2. In a large bowl, combine the salad greens, cherry tomatoes, cucumber, and red bell pepper. 3. In a small bowl, whisk together the olive oil and balsamic vinegar. Pour the dressing over the salad and toss to combine. 4. Top the salad with the sliced grilled chicken.

PER SERVING			
Calories: 350kcal	Fat: 15g	Carbs: 10g	Protein: 40g

Shrimp and Avocado Salad

PREPARATION TIME Min. 10	COOKING TIME Min. 10	SERVING 1

INGREDIENTS	DIRECTIONS
• 1 cup shrimp, peeled and deveined • 1 avocado, sliced • 2 cups mixed salad greens • 1/2 cup cherry tomatoes, halved • 1/4 cup red onion, thinly sliced • 1 tablespoon olive oil • 2 tablespoons lemon juice • Salt and pepper to taste	1. In a pan, heat 1 tablespoon of olive oil over medium heat. Add the shrimp and cook for 2-3 minutes on each side or until pink and opaque. Season with salt and pepper. 2. In a large bowl, combine the salad greens, cherry tomatoes, red onion, and avocado. 3. In a small bowl, whisk together the olive oil and lemon juice. Pour the dressing over the salad and toss to combine. 4. Top the salad with the cooked shrimp.

PER SERVING			
Calories: 400kcal	Fat: 25g	Carbs: 20g	Protein: 25g

Beef and Broccoli Stir-Fry

PREPARATION TIME	COOKING TIME	SERVING
Min. 10	Min. 15	1

INGREDIENTS	DIRECTIONS
• 1/2 pound beef sirloin, thinly sliced • 1 cup broccoli florets • 1/2 cup bell pepper, sliced • 1/4 cup soy sauce • 1 tablespoon olive oil • 1 teaspoon ginger, minced • 1 teaspoon garlic, minced • Salt and pepper to taste • 1 tablespoon sesame seeds	1. In a pan, heat the olive oil over medium heat. Add the ginger and garlic and cook for 1-2 minutes until fragrant. 2. Add the beef and cook for 3-4 minutes on each side or until cooked to your desired doneness. Remove the beef from the pan and set aside. 3. In the same pan, add the broccoli and bell pepper and cook for 5-7 minutes until tender. 4. Add the beef back to the pan and pour the soy sauce over the mixture. Stir well to combine. 5. Sprinkle with sesame seeds before serving.

PER SERVING			
Calories: 450kcal	Fat: 20g	Carbs: 15g	Protein: 50g

Turkey and Cheese Lettuce Wraps

PREPARATION TIME	COOKING TIME	SERVING
Min. 10	Min. 0	1

INGREDIENTS	DIRECTIONS
• 4 large lettuce leaves • 1/2 pound turkey breast, thinly sliced • 1/4 cup cheddar cheese, shredded • 1/4 cup cucumber, sliced • 1/4 cup red bell pepper, sliced • 1/4 cup mayonnaise • 1 tablespoon mustard • Salt and pepper to taste	1. Lay the lettuce leaves flat on a clean surface. 2. Spread a thin layer of mayonnaise and mustard on each lettuce leaf. 3. Top with turkey, cheese, cucumber, and bell pepper. Season with salt and pepper. 4. Roll up the lettuce leaves and secure with a toothpick if necessary.

PER SERVING			
Calories: 400kcal	Fat: 25g	Carbs: 10g	Protein: 35g

Chicken and Vegetable Skewers

PREPARATION TIME	COOKING TIME	SERVING
Min. 10	Min. 15	1

INGREDIENTS	DIRECTIONS
<ul><li>1 chicken breast, cut into cubes</li><li>1/2 cup bell pepper, cut into cubes</li><li>1/2 cup zucchini, cut into cubes</li><li>1/2 cup cherry tomatoes</li><li>1 tablespoon olive oil</li><li>1 teaspoon paprika</li><li>1 teaspoon garlic powder</li><li>Salt and pepper to taste</li></ul>	1. Preheat the grill to medium heat. 2. In a bowl, combine the olive oil, paprika, garlic powder, salt, and pepper. Add the chicken and vegetables and toss to coat. 3. Thread the chicken and vegetables onto skewers. 4. Grill the skewers for 6-7 minutes on each side or until the chicken is fully cooked.

PER SERVING

Calories: 350kcal	Fat: 115g	Carbs: 15g	Protein: 40g

Tuna Salad Stuffed Avocado

PREPARATION TIME	COOKING TIME	SERVING
Min. 10	Min. 0	1

INGREDIENTS	DIRECTIONS
<ul><li>1 avocado, halved and pitted</li><li>1 can (5 oz) tuna, drained</li><li>1/4 cup mayonnaise</li><li>1/4 cup celery, chopped</li><li>1/4 cup red onion, chopped</li><li>1 tablespoon lemon juice</li><li>Salt and pepper to taste</li><li>1 tablespoon chives, chopped</li></ul>	1. In a bowl, combine the tuna, mayonnaise, celery, red onion, lemon juice, salt, and pepper. 2. Scoop the tuna salad into the avocado halves. 3. Sprinkle with chives before serving.

PER SERVING

Calories: 450kcal	Fat: 35g	Carbs: 20g	Protein: 25g

Egg Salad Lettuce Wraps

PREPARATION TIME	COOKING TIME	SERVING
Min. 10	Min. 10	1

INGREDIENTS	DIRECTIONS
<ul><li>4 large lettuce leaves</li><li>4 eggs</li><li>1/4 cup mayonnaise</li><li>1 tablespoon mustard</li><li>1/4 cup celery, chopped</li><li>1/4 cup red onion, chopped</li><li>Salt and pepper to taste</li><li>1 tablespoon chives, chopped</li></ul>	1. Place the eggs in a saucepan and cover with water. Bring to a boil, then reduce the heat and simmer for 10 minutes. Drain and let cool. Peel and chop the eggs. 2. In a bowl, combine the chopped eggs, mayonnaise, mustard, celery, red onion, salt, and pepper. 3. Lay the lettuce leaves flat on a clean surface. Scoop the egg salad onto the lettuce leaves. 4. Roll up the lettuce leaves and secure with a toothpick if necessary.

5. Sprinkle with chives before serving.

PER SERVING			
Calories: 400kcal	Fat: 30g	Carbs: 10g	Protein: 20g

Turkey and Vegetable Roll-Ups

PREPARATION TIME	COOKING TIME	SERVING
Min. 10	Min. 0	1

INGREDIENTS	DIRECTIONS
• 1/2 pound turkey breast, thinly sliced • 1/4 cup cream cheese, softened • 1/4 cup cucumber, sliced • 1/4 cup red bell pepper, sliced • 1/4 cup spinach leaves • Salt and pepper to taste	1. Lay the turkey slices flat on a clean surface. 2. Spread a thin layer of cream cheese on each turkey slice. 3. Top with cucumber, bell pepper, and spinach. Season with salt and pepper. 4. Roll up the turkey slices and secure with a toothpick if necessary.

PER SERVING			
Calories: 350kcal	Fat: 20g	Carbs: 10g	Protein: 35g

Chicken and Avocado Salad

PREPARATION TIME	COOKING TIME	SERVING
Min. 10	Min. 15	1

INGREDIENTS	DIRECTIONS
• 1 chicken breast • 1 avocado, sliced • 2 cups mixed salad greens • 1/2 cup cherry tomatoes, halved • 1/4 cup red onion, thinly sliced • 1 tablespoon olive oil • 2 tablespoons lemon juice • Salt and pepper to taste	1. Season the chicken breast with salt and pepper. Grill the chicken breast for about 6-7 minutes on each side or until fully cooked. Slice the chicken into strips. 2. In a large bowl, combine the salad greens, cherry tomatoes, red onion, and avocado. 3. In a small bowl, whisk together the olive oil and lemon juice. Pour the dressing over the salad and toss to combine. 4. Top the salad with the sliced grilled chicken.

PER SERVING			
Calories: 400kcal	Fat: 25g	Carbs: 20g	Protein: 30g

Beef and Vegetable Salad

PREPARATION TIME	COOKING TIME	SERVING
Min. 10	Min. 15	1

INGREDIENTS	DIRECTIONS
• 1/2 pound beef sirloin, thinly sliced • 2 cups mixed salad greens • 1/2 cup cherry tomatoes, halved • 1/4 cup cucumber, sliced • 1/4 cup red bell pepper, sliced • 1 tablespoon olive oil • 2 tablespoons balsamic vinegar • Salt and pepper to taste	1. Season the beef with salt and pepper. Grill the beef for about 3-4 minutes on each side or until cooked to your desired doneness. Slice the beef into strips. 2. In a large bowl, combine the salad greens, cherry tomatoes, cucumber, and red bell pepper. 3. In a small bowl, whisk together the olive oil and balsamic vinegar. Pour the dressing over the salad and toss to combine. 4. Top the salad with the sliced grilled beef.

PER SERVING

Calories: 400kcal	Fat: 20g	Carbs: 10g	Protein: 40g

Shrimp and Vegetable Skewers

PREPARATION TIME Min. 10	COOKING TIME Min. 10	SERVING 1

INGREDIENTS	DIRECTIONS
• 1 cup shrimp, peeled and deveined • 1/2 cup bell pepper, cut into cubes • 1/2 cup zucchini, cut into cubes • 1/2 cup cherry tomatoes • 1 tablespoon olive oil • 1 teaspoon paprika • 1 teaspoon garlic powder • Salt and pepper to taste	1. Preheat the grill to medium heat. 2. In a bowl, combine the olive oil, paprika, garlic powder, salt, and pepper. Add the shrimp and vegetables and toss to coat. 3. Thread the shrimp and vegetables onto skewers. 4. Grill the skewers for 3-4 minutes on each side or until the shrimp is pink and opaque.

PER SERVING

Calories: 350kcal	Fat: 15g	Carbs: 15g	Protein: 35g

Tuna and Cucumber Roll-Ups

PREPARATION TIME Min. 10	COOKING TIME Min. 0	SERVING 1

INGREDIENTS	DIRECTIONS
• 1 can (5 oz) tuna, drained • 1/4 cup mayonnaise • 1 tablespoon lemon juice • 1/4 cup red onion, chopped • 1/4 cup celery, chopped • Salt and pepper to taste • 1 cucumber, thinly sliced lengthwise	1. In a bowl, combine the tuna, mayonnaise, lemon juice, red onion, celery, salt, and pepper. 2. Lay the cucumber slices flat on a clean surface. Scoop the tuna salad onto the cucumber slices.

3. Roll up the cucumber slices and secure with a toothpick if necessary.

PER SERVING			
Calories: 350kcal	Fat: 25g	Carbs: 10g	Protein: 25g

Chicken and Cheese Lettuce Wraps

PREPARATION TIME Min. 10	COOKING TIME Min. 15	SERVING 1

INGREDIENTS	DIRECTIONS
• 1 chicken breast, cut into strips • 4 large lettuce leaves • 1/4 cup cheddar cheese, shredded • 1/4 cup red bell pepper, sliced • 1/4 cup cucumber, sliced • 1 tablespoon olive oil • Salt and pepper to taste	1. In a pan, heat the olive oil over medium heat. Add the chicken and cook for 6-7 minutes on each side or until fully cooked. 2. Lay the lettuce leaves flat on a clean surface. Top with chicken, cheese, bell pepper, and cucumber. Season with salt and pepper. 3. Roll up the lettuce leaves and secure with a toothpick if necessary.

PER SERVING			
Calories: 350kcal	Fat: 10g	Carbs: 20g	Protein: 35g

Turkey and Avocado Salad

PREPARATION TIME Min. 10	COOKING TIME Min. 0	SERVING 1

INGREDIENTS	DIRECTIONS
• 1/2 pound turkey breast, thinly sliced • 1 avocado, sliced • 2 cups mixed salad greens • 1/2 cup cherry tomatoes, halved • 1/4 cup red onion, thinly sliced • 1 tablespoon olive oil • 2 tablespoons lemon juice • Salt and pepper to taste	1. In a large bowl, combine the salad greens, cherry tomatoes, red onion, and avocado. 2. In a small bowl, whisk together the olive oil and lemon juice. Pour the dressing over the salad and toss to combine. 3. Top the salad with the sliced turkey.

PER SERVING			
Calories: 350kcal	Fat: 20g	Carbs: 15g	Protein: 30g

Beef and Mushroom Skewers

PREPARATION TIME Min. 10	COOKING TIME Min. 15	SERVING 1

INGREDIENTS	DIRECTIONS
• 1/2 pound beef sirloin, cut into cubes • 1 cup mushrooms, halved • 1 tablespoon olive oil • 1 teaspoon garlic powder • 1 teaspoon paprika • Salt and pepper to taste	1. Preheat the grill to medium heat. 2. In a bowl, combine the olive oil, garlic powder, paprika, salt, and pepper. Add the beef and mushrooms and toss to coat. 3. Thread the beef and mushrooms onto skewers. 4. Grill the skewers for 5-6 minutes on each side or until the beef is cooked to your desired doneness.

PER SERVING

Calories: 400kcal	Fat: 20g	Carbs: 10g	Protein: 45g

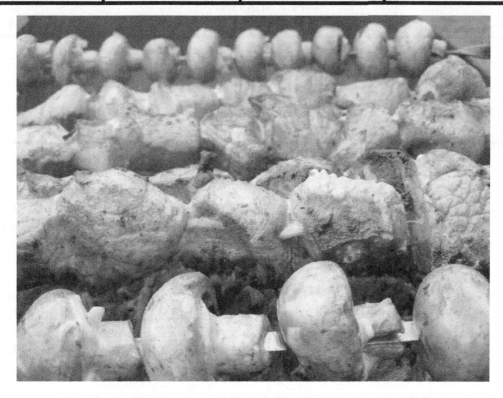

Delectable High-Carb Dinners

Spaghetti Squash with Tomato Sauce and Parmesan

PREPARATION TIME	COOKING TIME	SERVING
Min. 10	Min. 40	1

INGREDIENTS	DIRECTIONS
• 1 small spaghetti squash • 1 cup tomato sauce • 1/4 cup grated Parmesan cheese • 1 tablespoon olive oil • Salt and pepper to taste • 1 teaspoon dried basil • 1 teaspoon dried oregano	1. Preheat the oven to 400°F (200°C). 2. Cut the spaghetti squash in half lengthwise and remove the seeds. Drizzle with olive oil and season with salt and pepper.

3. Place the squash cut side down on a baking sheet and roast for 30-40 minutes or until tender.
4. While the squash is roasting, heat the tomato sauce in a saucepan over medium heat. Add the basil and oregano and simmer for 10 minutes.
5. Once the squash is done, use a fork to scrape the flesh into spaghetti-like strands.
6. Serve the squash with the tomato sauce and sprinkle with Parmesan cheese.

PER SERVING			
Calories: 350kcal	Fat: 15g	Carbs: 45g	Protein: 15g

Lentil and Vegetable Stuffed Bell Peppers

PREPARATION TIME	COOKING TIME	SERVING
Min. 15	Min. 45	1

INGREDIENTS	DIRECTIONS
<ul><li>1 large bell pepper</li><li>1/2 cup cooked lentils</li><li>1/2 cup cooked quinoa</li><li>1/2 cup diced tomatoes</li><li>1/4 cup diced red onion</li><li>1/4 cup shredded cheese</li><li>1 teaspoon olive oil</li><li>Salt and pepper to taste</li><li>1 teaspoon dried basil</li><li>1 teaspoon dried oregano</li></ul>	1. Preheat the oven to 375°F (190°C). 2. Cut the top off the bell pepper and remove the seeds and membranes. 3. In a bowl, combine the lentils, quinoa, tomatoes, onion, half of the cheese, olive oil, basil, oregano, salt, and pepper. 4. Stuff the bell pepper with the lentil mixture and place in a baking dish. 5. Sprinkle the remaining cheese on top. 6. Bake for 30-35 minutes or until the pepper is tender and the cheese is melted and bubbly.

PER SERVING			
Calories: 400kcal	Fat: 15g	Carbs: 50g	Protein: 20g

Sweet Potato and Chickpea Curry

PREPARATION TIME	COOKING TIME	SERVING
Min. 10	Min. 30	1

INGREDIENTS	DIRECTIONS
• 1 small sweet potato, peeled and diced • 1/2 cup canned chickpeas, drained and rinsed • 1 cup coconut milk • 1 tablespoon curry powder • 1/2 teaspoon turmeric • 1/2 teaspoon paprika • Salt and pepper to taste • 1 tablespoon olive oil • 2 cups spinach • Cooked brown rice for serving	1. In a large saucepan, heat the olive oil over medium heat. Add the sweet potato and cook for 5-7 minutes or until starting to soften. 2. Add the chickpeas, coconut milk, curry powder, turmeric, paprika, salt, and pepper. Bring to a boil, then reduce heat and simmer for 20-25 minutes or until the sweet potato is tender. 3. Stir in the spinach and cook until wilted. 4. Serve over cooked brown rice.

PER SERVING

Calories: 500kcal	Fat: 25g	Carbs: 60g	Protein: 15g

Vegetable and Bean Pasta

PREPARATION TIME Min. 10	COOKING TIME Min. 20	SERVING 1

INGREDIENTS	DIRECTIONS
• 1 cup cooked pasta • 1/2 cup canned cannellini beans, drained and rinsed • 1/2 cup diced tomatoes • 1/2 cup broccoli florets • 1/4 cup diced red onion • 1/4 cup grated Parmesan cheese • 1 tablespoon olive oil • Salt and pepper to taste • 1 teaspoon dried basil • 1 teaspoon dried oregano	1. In a large saucepan, heat the olive oil over medium heat. Add the onion and cook for 2-3 minutes or until softened. 2. Add the tomatoes, broccoli, beans, basil, oregano, salt, and pepper. Cook for 10-12 minutes or until the vegetables are tender. 3. Stir in the cooked pasta and heat through. 4. Serve with grated Parmesan cheese on top.

PER SERVING

Calories: 450kcal	Fat: 15g	Carbs: 60g	Protein: 20g

Quinoa and Vegetable Stir-Fry

PREPARATION TIME Min. 10	COOKING TIME Min. 15	SERVING 1

INGREDIENTS	DIRECTIONS
• 1/2 cup cooked quinoa • 1/2 cup broccoli florets • 1/2 cup sliced bell pepper • 1/2 cup sliced zucchini • 1/4 cup sliced red onion • 1/4 cup soy sauce • 1 tablespoon olive oil • 1 teaspoon sesame seeds • 1 teaspoon minced garlic • 1 teaspoon minced ginger	1. In a large pan, heat the olive oil over medium heat. Add the onion, bell pepper, zucchini, and broccoli and cook for 5-7 minutes or until the vegetables are tender. 2. Add the garlic and ginger and cook for another minute. 3. Stir in the cooked quinoa and soy sauce and heat through. 4. Serve sprinkled with sesame seeds.

PER SERVING

Calories: 400kcal	Fat: 15g	Carbs: 50g	Protein: 15g

Chickpea and Tomato Stew

PREPARATION TIME	COOKING TIME	SERVING
Min. 10	Min. 30	1

INGREDIENTS	DIRECTIONS
• 1/2 cup canned chickpeas, drained and rinsed • 1 cup diced tomatoes • 1/2 cup vegetable broth • 1/4 cup diced red onion • 1/4 cup chopped spinach • 1 tablespoon olive oil • Salt and pepper to taste • 1 teaspoon dried basil • 1 teaspoon dried oregano • Cooked brown rice for serving	1. In a large saucepan, heat the olive oil over medium heat. Add the onion and cook for 2-3 minutes or until softened. 2. Add the tomatoes, chickpeas, vegetable broth, basil, oregano, salt, and pepper. Bring to a boil, then reduce heat and simmer for 20-25 minutes or until the stew has thickened. 3. Stir in the spinach and cook until wilted. 4. Serve over cooked brown rice.

PER SERVING

Calories: 400kcal	Fat: 15g	Carbs: 55g	Protein: 15g

Creamy Pumpkin Soup

PREPARATION TIME	COOKING TIME	SERVING
Min. 10	Min. 30	1

INGREDIENTS	DIRECTIONS
• 1 cup pumpkin puree • 1 cup vegetable broth • 1/2 cup milk • 1/4 cup diced onion • 1 tablespoon butter • Salt and pepper to taste • 1 teaspoon dried thyme • 1 teaspoon dried sage	1. In a large saucepan, melt the butter over medium heat. Add the onion and cook for 2-3 minutes or until softened. 2. Add the pumpkin puree, vegetable broth, milk, thyme, sage, salt, and pepper. Bring to a boil, then reduce heat and simmer for 20-25 minutes. 3. Serve hot.

PER SERVING

Calories: 250kcal	Fat: 10g	Carbs: 35g	Protein: 5g

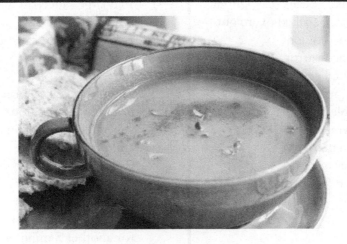

Vegetable Minestrone

PREPARATION TIME	COOKING TIME	SERVING
Min. 15	Min. 40	1

INGREDIENTS	DIRECTIONS
<ul><li>1/2 cup diced tomatoes</li><li>1/2 cup sliced carrots</li><li>1/2 cup sliced celery</li><li>1/2 cup chopped spinach</li><li>1/4 cup diced onion</li><li>1/4 cup canned cannellini beans, drained and rinsed</li><li>1 cup vegetable broth</li><li>1/2 cup small pasta</li><li>1 tablespoon olive oil</li><li>Salt and pepper to taste</li><li>1 teaspoon dried basil</li><li>1 teaspoon dried oregano</li></ul>	1. In a large saucepan, heat the olive oil over medium heat. Add the onion, carrots, and celery and cook for 5-7 minutes or until the vegetables are tender. 2. Add the tomatoes, beans, vegetable broth, basil, oregano, salt, and pepper. Bring to a boil, then reduce heat and simmer for 20-25 minutes. 3. Add the pasta and cook for an additional 10-12 minutes or until the pasta is tender. 4. Stir in the spinach and cook until wilted. 5. Serve hot.

PER SERVING

Calories: 350kcal	Fat: 10g	Carbs: 55g	Protein: 15g

Bean Soup

PREPARATION TIME	COOKING TIME	SERVING
Min. 10	1h	1

INGREDIENTS	DIRECTIONS
• 1 cup dried mixed beans (like kidney, black, pinto, etc.), soaked overnight • 1/2 cup chopped onion • 1/2 cup chopped carrot • 1/2 cup chopped celery • 2 cloves garlic, minced • 4 cups vegetable broth • 1 tsp dried thyme • 1 tsp dried rosemary • Salt and pepper to taste • 2 tbsp chopped fresh parsley • 1 tbsp olive oil	1. In a large saucepan, heat the olive oil over medium heat. 2. Add the onion, carrot, celery, and garlic and cook for 5-7 minutes until they start to soften. 3. Drain the soaked beans and add them to the saucepan along with the vegetable broth, thyme, rosemary, salt, and pepper. 4. Bring to a boil, then reduce the heat to low and simmer for about 1 hour until the beans are tender. 5. Stir in the chopped parsley and cook for another 5 minutes. 6. Serve immediately.

PER SERVING

Calories: 350kcal	Fat: 7g	Carbs: 55g	Protein: 20g

Pasta with Roasted Vegetables and Pesto

PREPARATION TIME	COOKING TIME	SERVING
Min. 10	Min. 30	1

INGREDIENTS	DIRECTIONS
• 1 cup cooked pasta • 1/2 cup sliced bell peppers • 1/2 cup sliced zucchini • 1/2 cup cherry tomatoes, halved • 1/4 cup sliced onion • 1/4 cup pesto sauce • 2 tablespoons olive oil • Salt and pepper to taste • 1 teaspoon dried basil • 1 teaspoon dried oregano	1. Preheat the oven to 400°F (200°C). 2. In a large bowl, combine the bell peppers, zucchini, tomatoes, onion, olive oil, basil, oregano, salt, and pepper. Toss well to combine. 3. Spread the vegetables on a baking sheet and roast for 20-25 minutes or until the vegetables are tender and slightly caramelized. 4. Stir the roasted vegetables and pesto sauce into the cooked pasta and heat through. 5. Serve hot.

PER SERVING

Calories: 550kcal	Fat: 25g	Carbs: 65g	Protein: 15g

Mushroom and Barley Soup

PREPARATION TIME	COOKING TIME	SERVING
Min. 15	Min. 45	1

INGREDIENTS

- 1/2 cup barley
- 1 cup sliced mushrooms
- 1/2 cup chopped onion
- 1/2 cup chopped carrot
- 1/2 cup chopped celery
- 4 cups vegetable broth
- 1 tbsp olive oil
- Salt and pepper to taste
- 2 tbsp chopped fresh parsley

DIRECTIONS

1. In a large saucepan, heat the olive oil over medium heat.
2. Add the onion, carrot, and celery and cook for 5-7 minutes until they start to soften.
3. Add the mushrooms and cook for another 5 minutes.
4. Add the barley, vegetable broth, salt, and pepper. Bring to a boil.
5. Reduce the heat to low and simmer for 30-35 minutes until the barley is tender.
6. Sprinkle with chopped parsley before serving.

PER SERVING

Calories: 350kcal	Fat: 10g	Carbs: 60g	Protein: 10g

Tomato Soup

PREPARATION TIME	COOKING TIME	SERVING
Min. 10	Min. 30	1

INGREDIENTS

- 4 large tomatoes, chopped
- 1/2 cup chopped onion
- 2 cloves garlic, minced
- 2 cups vegetable broth
- 1 tbsp olive oil
- 1 tsp sugar
- Salt and pepper to taste
- 2 tbsp chopped fresh basil
- 1/4 cup heavy cream (optional)

DIRECTIONS

1. In a large saucepan, heat the olive oil over medium heat.
2. Add the onion and garlic and cook for 5-7 minutes until they start to soften.
3. Add the tomatoes, vegetable broth, sugar, salt, and pepper. Bring to a boil.
4. Reduce the heat to low and simmer for 20-25 minutes until the tomatoes are tender.
5. Use an immersion blender to puree the soup until smooth. If you don't have an immersion blender, carefully transfer the soup to a blender and puree until smooth. Return the soup to the saucepan.
6. Stir in the chopped basil and heavy cream (if using). Heat the soup for another 2-3 minutes until it is heated through.
7. Serve immediately.

PER SERVING

Calories: 250kcal	Fat: 10g	Carbs: 35g	Protein: 5g

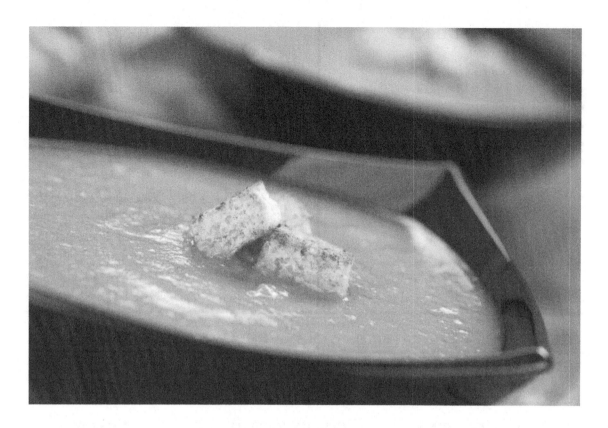

Savory Low-Carb Dinners

Lemon Garlic Roasted Chicken

PREPARATION TIME	COOKING TIME	SERVING
Min. 10	Min. 50	1

INGREDIENTS	DIRECTIONS
• 1 chicken breast • 2 tablespoons olive oil • 1 lemon, juiced • 3 cloves garlic, minced • 1 teaspoon dried thyme • Salt and pepper to taste	1. Preheat the oven to 400°F (200°C). 2. In a small bowl, mix together the olive oil, lemon juice, garlic, thyme, salt, and pepper. 3. Place the chicken breast in a baking dish and brush with the olive oil mixture. 4. Bake for 45-50 minutes or until the chicken is cooked through. 5. Serve immediately.

PER SERVING			
Calories: 350kcal	Fat: 20g	Carbs: 5g	Protein: 35g

Baked Salmon with Asparagus

PREPARATION TIME	COOKING TIME	SERVING
Min. 10	Min. 20	1

INGREDIENTS	DIRECTIONS
• 1 salmon fillet • 1 bunch asparagus, trimmed • 2 tablespoons olive oil • 1 lemon, juiced • 1 teaspoon minced garlic • Salt and pepper to taste	1. Preheat the oven to 400°F (200°C). 2. Place the salmon and asparagus on a baking sheet. 3. In a small bowl, mix together the olive oil, lemon juice, garlic, salt, and pepper. 4. Brush the salmon and asparagus with the olive oil mixture. 5. Bake for 15-20 minutes or until the salmon is cooked through and the asparagus is tender. 6. Serve immediately.

PER SERVING

Calories: 350kcal	Fat: 20g	Carbs: 10g	Protein: 35g

Beef Stir-Fry with Broccoli

PREPARATION TIME	COOKING TIME	SERVING
Min. 10	Min. 15	1

INGREDIENTS	DIRECTIONS
• 1/2 pound beef sirloin, thinly sliced • 1 cup broccoli florets • 1 tablespoon olive oil • 2 tablespoons soy sauce • 1 tablespoon oyster sauce • 1 teaspoon minced garlic • 1 teaspoon minced ginger • Salt and pepper to taste	1. Heat the olive oil in a pan over medium heat. 2. Add the garlic and ginger and cook for 1-2 minutes. 3. Add the beef and cook for 3-5 minutes or until browned. 4. Add the broccoli, soy sauce, oyster sauce, salt, and pepper and cook for another 5-7 minutes or until the broccoli is tender. 5. Serve immediately.

PER SERVING

Calories: 350kcal	Fat: 15g	Carbs: 15g	Protein: 40g

Pork Chops with Green Beans

PREPARATION TIME	COOKING TIME	SERVING
Min. 10	Min. 20	1

INGREDIENTS	DIRECTIONS
• 1 pork chop • 1 cup green beans, trimmed • 2 tablespoons olive oil • 1 tablespoon lemon juice • 1 teaspoon minced garlic • Salt and pepper to taste	1. Preheat the oven to 400°F (200°C). 2. Place the pork chop and green beans on a baking sheet. 3. In a small bowl, mix together the olive oil, lemon juice, garlic, salt, and pepper. 4. Brush the pork chop and green beans with the olive oil mixture.

5. Bake for 15-20 minutes or until the pork chop is cooked through and the green beans are tender.
6. Serve immediately.

PER SERVING			
Calories: 350kcal	Fat: 20g	Carbs: 10g	Protein: 35g

Shrimp Scampi with Zucchini Noodles

PREPARATION TIME Min. 10	COOKING TIME Min. 10	SERVING 1

INGREDIENTS	DIRECTIONS
• 1/2 pound shrimp, peeled and deveined • 1 zucchini, spiralized • 2 tablespoons olive oil • 1 lemon, juiced • 1 teaspoon minced garlic • 1/4 teaspoon red pepper flakes • Salt and pepper to taste	1. Heat the olive oil in a pan over medium heat. 2. Add the garlic and red pepper flakes and cook for 1-2 minutes. 3. Add the shrimp and cook for 3-5 minutes or until pink and opaque. 4. Add the zucchini noodles, lemon juice, salt, and pepper and cook for another 2-3 minutes or until the noodles are tender. 5. Serve immediately.

PER SERVING			
Calories: 350kcal	Fat: 20g	Carbs: 10g	Protein: 35g

Grilled Steak with Roasted Vegetables

PREPARATION TIME Min. 10	COOKING TIME Min. 20	SERVING 1

INGREDIENTS	DIRECTIONS
• 1 steak • 1 cup mixed vegetables (e.g., bell peppers, zucchini, cherry tomatoes) • 2 tablespoons olive oil • 1 teaspoon minced garlic • Salt and pepper to taste	1. Preheat the grill to medium-high heat. 2. In a small bowl, mix together the olive oil, garlic, salt, and pepper. 3. Brush the steak and vegetables with the olive oil mixture. 4. Grill the steak for 4-5 minutes on each side or until cooked to your desired doneness. 5. Grill the vegetables for 5-7 minutes or until tender. 6. Serve immediately.

PER SERVING			
Calories: 450kcal	Fat: 25g	Carbs: 15g	Protein: 40g

Baked Cod with Lemon and Dill

PREPARATION TIME Min. 10	COOKING TIME Min. 20	SERVING 1

INGREDIENTS	DIRECTIONS
• 1 cod fillet • 2 tablespoons olive oil • 1 lemon, juiced • 1 teaspoon dried dill • Salt and pepper to taste	1. Preheat the oven to 400°F (200°C). 2. Place the cod fillet on a baking sheet. 3. In a small bowl, mix together the olive oil, lemon juice, dill, salt, and pepper. 4. Brush the cod fillet with the olive oil mixture. 5. Bake for 15-20 minutes or until the cod is cooked through. 6. Serve immediately.

PER SERVING			
Calories: 250kcal	Fat: 15g	Carbs: 5g	Protein: 25g

Chicken Fajitas with Bell Peppers and Onions

PREPARATION TIME Min. 10	COOKING TIME Min. 15	SERVING 1

INGREDIENTS	DIRECTIONS
• 1 chicken breast, thinly sliced • 1 bell pepper, thinly sliced • 1 onion, thinly sliced • 2 tablespoons olive oil • 1 teaspoon chili powder • 1 teaspoon cumin • 1 teaspoon paprika • Salt and pepper to taste	1. Heat the olive oil in a pan over medium heat. 2. Add the chicken and cook for 3-5 minutes or until browned. 3. Add the bell pepper, onion, chili powder, cumin, paprika, salt, and pepper and cook for another 5-7 minutes or until the vegetables are tender. 4. Serve immediately.

PER SERVING			
Calories: 350kcal	Fat: 15g	Carbs: 15g	Protein: 35g

Pork Tenderloin with Roasted Brussels Sprouts

PREPARATION TIME Min. 10	COOKING TIME Min. 25	SERVING 1

INGREDIENTS	DIRECTIONS
• 1 pork tenderloin • 1 cup Brussels sprouts, halved • 2 tablespoons olive oil • 1 teaspoon minced garlic • Salt and pepper to taste	1. Preheat the oven to 400°F (200°C). 2. Place the pork tenderloin and Brussels sprouts on a baking sheet. 3. In a small bowl, mix together the olive oil, garlic, salt, and pepper.

4. Brush the pork tenderloin and Brussels sprouts with the olive oil mixture.
5. Bake for 20-25 minutes or until the pork tenderloin is cooked through and the Brussels sprouts are tender.
6. Serve immediately.

PER SERVING			
Calories: 350kcal	Fat: 15g	Carbs: 15g	Protein: 35g

Grilled Shrimp with Garlic and Herbs

PREPARATION TIME	COOKING TIME	SERVING
Min. 10	Min. 10	1

INGREDIENTS	DIRECTIONS
• 1/2 pound shrimp, peeled and deveined • 2 tablespoons olive oil • 1 teaspoon minced garlic • 1 teaspoon dried herbs (e.g., thyme, rosemary, oregano) • Salt and pepper to taste	1. Preheat the grill to medium-high heat. 2. In a small bowl, mix together the olive oil, garlic, herbs, salt, and pepper. 3. Thread the shrimp onto skewers and brush with the olive oil mixture. 4. Grill for 3-5 minutes on each side or until the shrimp are pink and opaque. 5. Serve immediately.

PER SERVING			
Calories: 250kcal	Fat: 15g	Carbs: 5g	Protein: 25g

Beef and Vegetable Kebabs

PREPARATION TIME	COOKING TIME	SERVING
Min. 10	Min. 10	1

INGREDIENTS	DIRECTIONS
• 1/2 pound beef sirloin, cut into cubes • 1 bell pepper, cut into chunks • 1 onion, cut into chunks • 2 tablespoons olive oil • 1 teaspoon minced garlic • Salt and pepper to taste	1. Preheat the grill to medium-high heat. 2. Thread the beef, bell pepper, and onion onto skewers. 3. In a small bowl, mix together the olive oil, garlic, salt, and pepper. 4. Brush the kebabs with the olive oil mixture. 5. Grill for 3-5 minutes on each side or until the beef is cooked to your desired doneness and the vegetables are tender. 6. Serve immediately.

PER SERVING			
Calories: 350kcal	Fat: 15g	Carbs: 15g	Protein: 35g

Chicken and Vegetable Stir-Fry

PREPARATION TIME Min. 10	COOKING TIME Min. 15	SERVING 1

INGREDIENTS	DIRECTIONS
• 1 chicken breast, thinly sliced • 1 cup mixed vegetables (e.g., bell peppers, broccoli, carrots) • 2 tablespoons olive oil • 2 tablespoons soy sauce • 1 teaspoon minced garlic • 1 teaspoon minced ginger • Salt and pepper to taste	1. Heat the olive oil in a pan over medium heat. 2. Add the garlic and ginger and cook for 1-2 minutes. 3. Add the chicken and cook for 3-5 minutes or until browned. 4. Add the vegetables, soy sauce, salt, and pepper and cook for another 5-7 minutes or until the vegetables are tender. 5. Serve immediately.

PER SERVING			
Calories: 350kcal	Fat: 15g	Carbs: 15g	Protein: 35g

Pork Chops with Roasted Vegetables

PREPARATION TIME Min. 10	COOKING TIME Min. 20	SERVING 1

INGREDIENTS	DIRECTIONS
• 1 pork chop • 1 cup mixed vegetables (e.g., bell peppers, zucchini, cherry tomatoes) • 2 tablespoons olive oil • 1 teaspoon minced garlic • Salt and pepper to taste	1. Preheat the oven to 400°F (200°C). 2. Place the pork chop and vegetables on a baking sheet. 3. In a small bowl, mix together the olive oil, garlic, salt, and pepper. 4. Brush the pork chop and vegetables with the olive oil mixture. 5. Bake for 15-20 minutes or until the pork chop is cooked through and the vegetables are tender. 6. Serve immediately.

PER SERVING			
Calories: 350kcal	Fat: 20g	Carbs: 15g	Protein: 35g

Baked Tilapia with Lemon and Herbs

PREPARATION TIME Min. 10	COOKING TIME Min. 20	SERVING 1

INGREDIENTS	DIRECTIONS
• 1 tilapia fillet • 2 tablespoons olive oil • 1 lemon, juiced	1. Preheat the oven to 400°F (200°C). 2. Place the tilapia fillet on a baking sheet.

- 1 teaspoon dried herbs (e.g., thyme, rosemary, oregano)
- Salt and pepper to taste

3. In a small bowl, mix together the olive oil, lemon juice, herbs, salt, and pepper.
4. Brush the tilapia fillet with the olive oil mixture.
5. Bake for 15-20 minutes or until the tilapia is cooked through.
6. Serve immediately.

PER SERVING			
Calories: 250kcal	Fat: 15g	Carbs: 5g	Protein: 25g

Beef and Mushroom Stir-Fry

PREPARATION TIME Min. 10	COOKING TIME Min. 15	SERVING 1

INGREDIENTS	DIRECTIONS
<ul><li>1/2 pound beef sirloin, thinly sliced</li><li>1 cup mushrooms, sliced</li><li>2 tablespoons olive oil</li><li>2 tablespoons soy sauce</li><li>1 teaspoon minced garlic</li><li>1 teaspoon minced ginger</li><li>Salt and pepper to taste</li></ul>	1. Heat the olive oil in a pan over medium heat. 2. Add the garlic and ginger and cook for 1-2 minutes. 3. Add the beef and cook for 3-5 minutes or until browned. 4. Add the mushrooms, soy sauce, salt, and pepper and cook for another 5-7 minutes or until the mushrooms are tender. 5. Serve immediately.

PER SERVING			
Calories: 350kcal	Fat: 15g	Carbs: 10g	Protein: 35g

Chicken and Asparagus Stir-Fry

PREPARATION TIME Min. 10	COOKING TIME Min. 15	SERVING 1

INGREDIENTS	DIRECTIONS
<ul><li>1 chicken breast, thinly sliced</li><li>1 cup asparagus, chopped</li><li>2 tablespoons olive oil</li><li>2 tablespoons soy sauce</li><li>1 teaspoon minced garlic</li><li>1 teaspoon minced ginger</li><li>Salt and pepper to taste</li></ul>	1. Heat the olive oil in a pan over medium heat. 2. Add the garlic and ginger and cook for 1-2 minutes. 3. Add the chicken and cook for 3-5 minutes or until browned. 4. Add the asparagus, soy sauce, salt, and pepper and cook for another 5-7 minutes or until the asparagus is tender. 5. Serve immediately.

PER SERVING			
Calories: 350kcal	Fat: 15g	Carbs: 10g	Protein: 35g

Spicy Shrimp and Cauliflower Rice

PREPARATION TIME Min. 10	COOKING TIME Min. 15	SERVING 1

INGREDIENTS	DIRECTIONS
• 1 cup cauliflower rice • 1/2 pound shrimp, peeled and deveined • 1 tablespoon olive oil • 1 teaspoon chili flakes • 1 teaspoon minced garlic • Salt and pepper to taste • 2 tablespoons chopped fresh cilantro	1. Heat the olive oil in a pan over medium heat. 2. Add the garlic and chili flakes and cook for 1-2 minutes. 3. Add the shrimp and cook for 3-5 minutes or until pink and cooked through. 4. Add the cauliflower rice, salt, and pepper and cook for another 5-7 minutes or until the cauliflower rice is tender. 5. Stir in the cilantro. 6. Serve immediately.

PER SERVING			
Calories: 350kcal	Fat: 15g	Carbs: 10g	Protein: 35g

Snacks, Smoothies, and Quick Bites

Apple and Almond Butter Sandwich

PREPARATION TIME Min. 5	COOKING TIME Min. 0	SERVING 1

INGREDIENTS	DIRECTIONS
• 1 apple, sliced • 2 tablespoons almond butter • 1 tablespoon honey • 1 teaspoon cinnamon	1. Spread the almond butter on one side of each apple slice. 2. Drizzle the honey and sprinkle the cinnamon over the almond butter. 3. Top with another apple slice to make a sandwich. 4. Repeat with the remaining apple slices.

PER SERVING			
Calories: 320kcal	Fat: 18g	Carbs: 40g	Protein: 6g

Berry and Banana Smoothie Preparation

PREPARATION TIME Min. 5	COOKING TIME Min. 0	SERVING 1

INGREDIENTS	DIRECTIONS
• 1 banana • 1 cup mixed berries • 1 cup almond milk	1. Place all the ingredients in a blender. 2. Blend until smooth. 3. Serve immediately.

- 1 tablespoon honey

PER SERVING			
Calories: 250kcal	Fat: 3g	Carbs: 55g	Protein: 3g

Peanut Butter and Jelly Energy Bites

PREPARATION TIME Min. 10	COOKING TIME Min. 0	SERVING 1

INGREDIENTS	DIRECTIONS
• 1 cup oats • 1/2 cup peanut butter • 1/4 cup jelly • 1 tablespoon chia seeds • 1 tablespoon honey	1. In a bowl, mix all the ingredients until well combined. 2. Roll the mixture into 1-inch balls. 3. Place the balls on a tray lined with parchment paper. 4. Refrigerate for at least 1 hour before serving.

PER SERVING			
Calories: 450kcal	Fat: 24g	Carbs: 50g	Protein: 12g

Chocolate and Banana Smoothie

PREPARATION TIME Min. 5	COOKING TIME Min. 0	SERVING 1

INGREDIENTS	DIRECTIONS
• 1 banana • 1 cup almond milk • 1 tablespoon cocoa powder • 1 tablespoon honey	1. Place all the ingredients in a blender. 2. Blend until smooth. 3. Serve immediately.

PER SERVING			
Calories: 250kcal	Fat: 4g	Carbs: 55g	Protein: 3g

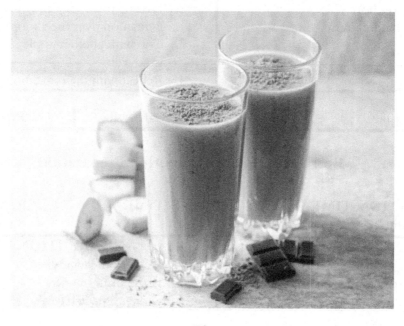

Trail Mix

PREPARATION TIME Min. 5	COOKING TIME Min. 0	SERVING 1

INGREDIENTS	DIRECTIONS
• 1/4 cup almonds • 1/4 cup walnuts • 1/4 cup dried cranberries • 1/4 cup dark chocolate chips	1. In a bowl, mix all the ingredients. 2. Store in an airtight container.

PER SERVING			
Calories: 450kcal	Fat: 30g	Carbs: 40g	Protein: 10g

Fruit and Nut Bars

PREPARATION TIME Min. 10	COOKING TIME Min. 0	SERVING 1

INGREDIENTS	DIRECTIONS
• 1 cup dates, pitted • 1/2 cup almonds • 1/2 cup dried cranberries • 1/4 cup shredded coconut	1. Place all the ingredients in a food processor. 2. Process until the mixture sticks together. 3. Press the mixture into a lined baking dish. 4. Refrigerate for at least 1 hour before cutting into bars.

PER SERVING			
Calories: 400kcal	Fat: 20g	Carbs: 50g	Protein: 8g

Oatmeal and Raisin Energy Bites

PREPARATION TIME Min. 10	COOKING TIME Min. 0	SERVING 1

INGREDIENTS	DIRECTIONS
• 1 cup oats • 1/2 cup peanut butter • 1/4 cup honey • 1/2 cup raisins • 1 teaspoon cinnamon	1. In a bowl, mix all the ingredients until well combined. 2. Roll the mixture into 1-inch balls. 3. Place the balls on a tray lined with parchment paper. 4. Refrigerate for at least 1 hour before serving.

PER SERVING			
Calories: 450kcal	Fat: 24g	Carbs: 50g	Protein: 12g

Cucumber and Hummus Roll-Ups

PREPARATION TIME	COOKING TIME	SERVING
Min. 10	Min. 0	1

INGREDIENTS	DIRECTIONS
• 1 cucumber • 1/4 cup hummus • 1/4 cup red bell pepper, thinly sliced • 1/4 cup carrot, thinly sliced	1. Slice the cucumber lengthwise into thin strips using a vegetable peeler. 2. Spread a thin layer of hummus on each cucumber strip. 3. Place the bell pepper and carrot slices at one end of the cucumber strip. 4. Roll the cucumber strip around the vegetables. 5. Repeat with the remaining cucumber strips and vegetables. 6. Serve immediately.

PER SERVING			
Calories: 150kcal	Fat: 8g	Carbs: 18g	Protein: 5g

Almond and Coconut Energy Bites

PREPARATION TIME	COOKING TIME	SERVING
Min. 10	Min. 0	1

INGREDIENTS	DIRECTIONS
• 1/2 cup almonds • 1/2 cup shredded coconut • 1/4 cup almond butter • 2 tablespoons honey	1. In a food processor, process the almonds until finely chopped. 2. Add the shredded coconut, almond butter, and honey. Process until the mixture sticks together. 3. Roll the mixture into 1-inch balls. 4. Place the balls on a tray lined with parchment paper. 5. Refrigerate for at least 1 hour before serving.

PER SERVING			
Calories: 400kcal	Fat: 35g	Carbs: 20g	Protein: 10g

Avocado and Tomato Salsa

PREPARATION TIME	COOKING TIME	SERVING
Min. 10	Min. 0	1

INGREDIENTS	DIRECTIONS
• 1 avocado, diced • 1 tomato, diced • 1/4 cup red onion, diced • 1 tablespoon lime juice • Salt and pepper, to taste	1. In a bowl, mix the avocado, tomato, and red onion. 2. Add the lime juice, salt, and pepper. Mix well.

3. Serve immediately with vegetable sticks or low-carb crackers.

| Calories: 250kcal | Fat: 20g | Carbs: 20g | Protein: 3g |

Berry and Chia Seed Pudding

PREPARATION TIME	COOKING TIME	SERVING
Min. 5	Min. 0	1

INGREDIENTS	DIRECTIONS
• 1 cup almond milk • 1/4 cup chia seeds • 1 tablespoon honey • 1/2 cup mixed berries	1. In a bowl, mix the almond milk, chia seeds, and honey. 2. Refrigerate for at least 4 hours or overnight until the chia seeds have absorbed the liquid and formed a pudding-like consistency. 3. Top with mixed berries before serving.

PER SERVING

| Calories: 300kcal | Fat: 15g | Carbs: 35g | Protein: 10g |

Cheese and Vegetable Sticks

PREPARATION TIME	COOKING TIME	SERVING
Min. 10	Min. 0	1

INGREDIENTS	DIRECTIONS
• 1/4 cup cheddar cheese, cut into sticks • 1/4 cup cucumber, cut into sticks • 1/4 cup bell pepper, cut into sticks • 1/4 cup carrot, cut into sticks	1. Arrange the cheese and vegetable sticks on a plate. 2. Serve with a side of low-carb dip or dressing.

PER SERVING

| Calories: 200kcal | Fat: 15g | Carbs: 10g | Protein: 10g |

Nut and Seed Mix

PREPARATION TIME	COOKING TIME	SERVING
Min. 5	Min. 0	1

INGREDIENTS	DIRECTIONS
• 1/4 cup almonds • 1/4 cup walnuts • 1/4 cup pumpkin seeds • 1/4 cup sunflower seeds	1. In a bowl, mix all the ingredients. 2. Store in an airtight container.

PER SERVING

| Calories: 450kcal | Fat: 40g | Carbs: 15g | Protein: 15g |

Chocolate and Almond Smoothie

PREPARATION TIME Min. 5	COOKING TIME Min. 0	SERVING 1

INGREDIENTS	DIRECTIONS
• 1 cup almond milk • 1 tablespoon cocoa powder • 1 tablespoon almond butter • 1 tablespoon chia seeds • 1 tablespoon honey	1. Place all the ingredients in a blender. 2. Blend until smooth. 3. Serve immediately.

PER SERVING			
Calories: 350kcal	Fat: 25g	Carbs: 30g	Protein: 10g

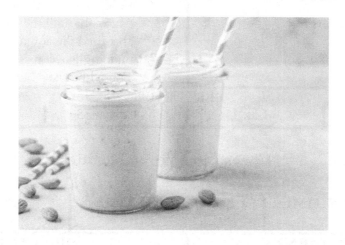

Guilt-Free Desserts for Every Carb Cycle

Baked Apple with Cinnamon

PREPARATION TIME Min. 10	COOKING TIME Min. 30	SERVING 1

INGREDIENTS	DIRECTIONS
• 1 large apple • 1 teaspoon cinnamon • 1 tablespoon honey • 2 tablespoons oats	1. Preheat the oven to 350°F (175°C). 2. Core the apple and place it on a baking sheet. 3. In a small bowl, mix the cinnamon, honey, and oats. 4. Stuff the apple with the oat mixture. 5. Bake for 30-35 minutes until the apple is tender. 6. Serve warm.

PER SERVING			
Calories: 200kcal	Fat: 1g	Carbs: 50g	Protein: 2g

Chocolate and Banana Mug Cake

PREPARATION TIME	COOKING TIME	SERVING
Min. 5	Min. 2	1

INGREDIENTS	DIRECTIONS
• 1 ripe banana, mashed • 2 tablespoons cocoa powder • 3 tablespoons oats • 1 tablespoon honey • 1/2 teaspoon baking powder	1. In a mug, mix the banana, cocoa powder, oats, honey, and baking powder. 2. Microwave on high for 2 minutes. 3. Let it cool for a few minutes before eating.

PER SERVING

Calories: 300kcal	Fat: 3g	Carbs: 70g	Protein: 7g

Berry and Yogurt Parfait

PREPARATION TIME	COOKING TIME	SERVING
Min. 5	Min. 0	1

INGREDIENTS	DIRECTIONS
• 1 cup mixed berries • 1 cup low-fat yogurt • 2 tablespoons granola • 1 tablespoon honey	1. In a glass, layer half of the berries, half of the yogurt, and half of the granola. 2. Drizzle with half of the honey. 3. Repeat the layers with the remaining ingredients. 4. Serve immediately.

PER SERVING

Calories: 350kcal	Fat: 5g	Carbs: 70g	Protein: 15g

Oatmeal and Peanut Butter Cookies

PREPARATION TIME	COOKING TIME	SERVING
Min. 10	Min. 12	1

INGREDIENTS	DIRECTIONS
• 1/2 cup oats • 2 tablespoons peanut butter • 1 tablespoon honey • 1/2 teaspoon baking powder • 1/4 cup dark chocolate chips	1. Preheat the oven to 350°F (175°C). 2. In a bowl, mix the oats, peanut butter, honey, and baking powder. 3. Fold in the chocolate chips. 4. Scoop tablespoon-sized portions of the dough onto a baking sheet lined with parchment paper. 5. Bake for 10-12 minutes until the edges are golden. 6. Let them cool before serving.

PER SERVING

Calories: 400kcal	Fat: 20g	Carbs: 50g	Protein: 10g

Pineapple and Coconut Sorbet

PREPARATION TIME Min. 10	COOKING TIME Min. 0	SERVING 1

INGREDIENTS	DIRECTIONS
• 1 cup pineapple, frozen • 1/2 cup coconut milk • 2 tablespoons honey	1. In a blender, blend the pineapple, coconut milk, and honey until smooth. 2. Transfer to a container and freeze for at least 2 hours. 3. Serve cold.

PER SERVING			
Calories: 300kcal	Fat: 10g	Carbs: 55g	Protein: 2g

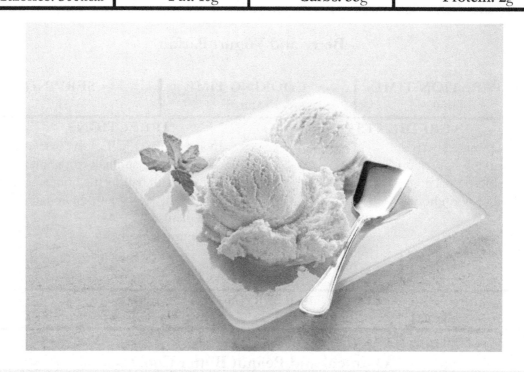

Chocolate and Avocado Mousse

PREPARATION TIME Min. 10	COOKING TIME Min. 0	SERVING 1

INGREDIENTS	DIRECTIONS
• 1 ripe avocado • 2 tablespoons cocoa powder • 2 tablespoons honey • 1/2 teaspoon vanilla extract	1. In a blender, blend the avocado, cocoa powder, honey, and vanilla extract until smooth. 2. Transfer to a bowl and refrigerate for at least 1 hour. 3. Serve cold.

PER SERVING			
Calories: 350kcal	Fat: 20g	Carbs: 45g	Protein: 5g

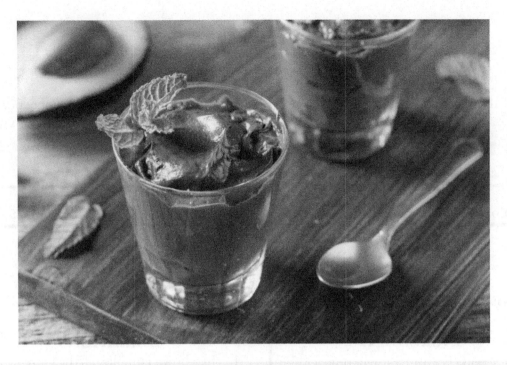

Apple and Cinnamon Muffins

PREPARATION TIME	COOKING TIME	SERVING
Min. 10	Min. 20	1

INGREDIENTS	DIRECTIONS
<ul><li>1/2 cup whole wheat flour</li><li>1/2 teaspoon baking powder</li><li>1/4 teaspoon baking soda</li><li>1/2 teaspoon cinnamon</li><li>1/4 cup apple sauce</li><li>2 tablespoons honey</li><li>1/4 cup milk</li><li>1/2 apple, diced</li></ul>	1. Preheat the oven to 350°F (175°C). 2. In a bowl, mix the flour, baking powder, baking soda, and cinnamon. 3. In another bowl, mix the apple sauce, honey, and milk. 4. Add the wet ingredients to the dry ingredients and mix until combined. 5. Fold in the diced apple. 6. Divide the batter into muffin cups lined with paper liners. 7. Bake for 18-20 minutes until a toothpick inserted into the center comes out clean. 8. Let them cool before serving.

PER SERVING			
Calories: 300kcal	Fat: 2g	Carbs: 70g	Protein: 5g

Berry Protein Gelato

PREPARATION TIME	COOKING TIME	SERVING
Min. 10	Min. 0	1

INGREDIENTS

- 1 cup mixed berries (frozen)
- 1 scoop vanilla protein powder
- 1/2 cup unsweetened almond milk
- 1 tbsp erythritol

DIRECTIONS

1. In a blender, combine all the ingredients.
2. Blend until smooth.
3. Transfer the mixture to a container and freeze for at least 4 hours or until firm.
4. Scoop the gelato into a bowl and serve.

PER SERVING			
Calories: 200kcal	Fat: 3g	Carbs: 20g	Protein: 25g

Protein Chocolate Pudding

PREPARATION TIME	COOKING TIME	SERVING
Min. 5	Min. 0	1

INGREDIENTS

- 1 scoop chocolate protein powder
- 1 cup Greek yogurt (non-fat)
- 1 tbsp cocoa powder
- 1 tbsp erythritol

DIRECTIONS

1. In a bowl, combine all the ingredients.
2. Mix until smooth.
3. Transfer the pudding to a serving bowl and refrigerate for at least 1 hour before serving.

PER SERVING			
Calories: 250kcal	Fat: 3g	Carbs: 15g	Protein: 40g

Protein Cheesecake Bites

PREPARATION TIME	COOKING TIME	SERVING
Min. 10	Min. 20	1

INGREDIENTS

- 1/2 cup cottage cheese (low-fat)
- 1 scoop vanilla protein powder
- 1 egg white
- 1 tbsp erythritol
- 1/2 tsp vanilla extract

DIRECTIONS

1. Preheat the oven to 350°F (175°C) and line a muffin tin with paper liners.
2. In a blender, combine all the ingredients.
3. Blend until smooth.
4. Divide the batter among the muffin cups.
5. Bake for 20-25 minutes or until the edges are golden and the center is set.
6. Remove from the oven and let it cool completely before serving.

PER SERVING			
Calories: 200kcal	Fat: 2g	Carbs: 10g	Protein: 30g

Protein Chocolate Chip Cookies

PREPARATION TIME	COOKING TIME	SERVING
Min.	Min.	1

INGREDIENTS	DIRECTIONS
• 1 cup almond flour • 1 scoop vanilla protein powder • 1/4 cup erythritol • 1/2 tsp baking powder • 1/4 cup unsweetened applesauce • 1 egg white • 1/2 tsp vanilla extract • 1/4 cup sugar-free chocolate chips	1. Preheat the oven to 350°F (175°C) and line a baking tray with parchment paper. 2. In a bowl, combine almond flour, protein powder, erythritol, and baking powder. 3. In another bowl, combine applesauce, egg white, and vanilla extract. 4. Add the wet ingredients to the dry ingredients and mix until a dough forms. 5. Fold in the chocolate chips. 6. Scoop tablespoon-sized portions of the dough onto the prepared baking tray. 7. Bake for 12-15 minutes or until the edges are golden. 8. Remove from the oven and let it cool completely before serving.

PER SERVING

Calories: 300kcal	Fat: 15g	Carbs: 15g	Protein: 25g

Protein Lemon Bars

PREPARATION TIME	COOKING TIME	SERVING
Min. 20	Min. 20	1

INGREDIENTS

- 1 cup almond flour
- 1/4 cup erythritol
- 1/4 cup unsweetened applesauce
- 1/2 tsp vanilla extract
- 3 egg whites
- 1/2 cup lemon juice
- 1 scoop vanilla protein powder
- 1/4 cup erythritol

DIRECTIONS

1. Preheat the oven to 350°F (175°C) and line a baking dish with parchment paper.
2. In a bowl, combine almond flour, 1/4 cup erythritol, applesauce, and vanilla extract.
3. Press the mixture into the bottom of the prepared baking dish.
4. Bake for 10-12 minutes or until the edges are golden.
5. In another bowl, whisk together egg whites, lemon juice, protein powder, and 1/4 cup erythritol.
6. Pour the mixture over the baked crust.
7. Bake for another 10-12 minutes or until the filling is set.
8. Remove from the oven and let it cool completely before serving.

PER SERVING

Calories: 350kcal	Fat: 15g	Carbs: 20g	Protein: 30g

Protein-Packed Peanut Butter Cups

PREPARATION TIME	COOKING TIME	SERVING
Min. 10	Min. 0	1

INGREDIENTS

- 1/4 cup peanut butter (unsweetened)
- 1 scoop chocolate protein powder
- 1 tbsp cocoa powder
- 1 tbsp erythritol
- 2 tbsp water

DIRECTIONS

1. In a bowl, combine peanut butter, protein powder, cocoa powder, erythritol, and water.
2. Mix until a dough forms.
3. Divide the dough into small portions and shape them into cups.
4. Place the cups on a tray lined with parchment paper and freeze for at least 1 hour before serving.

PER SERVING

Calories: 300kcal	Fat: 15g	Carbs: 10g	Protein: 30g

Protein-Packed Strawberry Cheesecake

PREPARATION TIME	COOKING TIME	SERVING
Min. 10	Min. 0	1

INGREDIENTS	DIRECTIONS
• 1/2 cup cottage cheese (low-fat) • 1 scoop vanilla protein powder • 1/2 cup strawberries (frozen) • 1 tbsp erythritol	1. In a blender, combine all the ingredients. 2. Blend until smooth. 3. Transfer the mixture to a serving bowl and refrigerate for at least 1 hour before serving.

PER SERVING			
Calories: 250kcal	Fat: 2g	Carbs: 20g	Protein: 35g

Protein-Packed Chocolate Cake

PREPARATION TIME Min. 10	COOKING TIME Min. 20	SERVING 1

INGREDIENTS	DIRECTIONS
• 1/2 cup almond flour • 1 scoop chocolate protein powder • 1/4 cup erythritol • 1/4 cup unsweetened applesauce • 1 egg white • 1/2 tsp baking powder • 1/4 cup water	1. Preheat the oven to 350°F (175°C) and grease a small cake tin. 2. In a bowl, combine all the ingredients. 3. Mix until smooth. 4. Pour the batter into the prepared cake tin. 5. Bake for 20-25 minutes or until a toothpick inserted into the center comes out clean. 6. Remove from the oven and let it cool completely before serving.

PER SERVING			
Calories: 350kcal	Fat: 15g	Carbs: 15g	Protein: 35g

Protein-Packed Vanilla Ice Cream

PREPARATION TIME Min. 10	COOKING TIME Min. 0	SERVING 1

INGREDIENTS	DIRECTIONS
• 1 cup Greek yogurt (non-fat) • 1 scoop vanilla protein powder • 1/4 cup erythritol • 1/2 tsp vanilla extract	1. In a bowl, combine all the ingredients. 2. Mix until smooth. 3. Transfer the mixture to an ice cream maker and churn according to the manufacturer's instructions. 4. Transfer the ice cream to a container and freeze for at least 4 hours or until firm. 5. Scoop the ice cream into a bowl and serve.

PER SERVING			
Calories: 250kcal	Fat: 2g	Carbs: 15g	Protein: 40g

Chapter 7: Personalizing Carb-Cycling for Your Goals

Starting a carb-cycling voyage is like to setting sail on wide, undiscovered waters. While the horizon promises transformation and happiness, the journey demands direction. The compass in Chapter 7, "Personalizing Carb-Cycling for Your Goals," will guide you through the complexities of personalizing this dietary strategy to your own needs, aspirations, and circumstances. This chapter goes further into making carb-cycling work for you, whether you're going for muscle definition, athletic prowess, or simply a healthier version of yourself. From understanding the physics behind weight plateaus to leveraging the power of carbs for specific demographics, we'll look at all the different ways you can make this journey uniquely yours.

Weight Loss and Fat Burning Focus

The popularity of weight reduction has resulted in a plethora of diets and exercise regimens, with carb-cycling emerging as a promising alternative, particularly for individuals experiencing weight loss plateaus or the boredom of restrictive diets. Carb-cycling, a regimen that involves alternating high-carb and low-carb days, tackles a variety of weight-loss aspects, ranging from metabolism to hormone balance. It manipulates carbs, the body's principal energy source, and their conversion into glucose and fat to speed up metabolism and push the body to burn stored fat. This method not only deceives the body, but also recognizes and works with its flexibility to prevent metabolic slowdown and energy conservation, which are typical causes of weight loss plateaus. It promotes fat loss while keeping or growing muscle, rather than just weight loss, which can involve water, muscle, or fat loss. This is critical since muscles are metabolically active and burn calories even while resting. Furthermore, carb-cycling enhances insulin sensitivity, which is necessary for controlling blood sugar levels and is frequently affected by recurrent carbohydrate overconsumption, leading to insulin resistance, an increased risk of type 2 diabetes, and weight loss issues. Carb-cycling improves insulin response and facilitates weight and fat loss by changing carb consumption. Finally, carb-cycling is more than just a trendy diet; it is a deliberate method based on the body's metabolic workings for optimal weight and fat loss. It provides a new, scientifically informed perspective for those who have been frustrated by existing diets and are battling with weight loss. It stresses working with the body and recognizes the mental and physical sides of weight loss, where consistency, adaptation, and metabolic manipulation can result in revolutionary results.

Muscle Building and Athletic Performance

While losing weight is a frequent fitness goal, many people also want to gain lean muscle mass and improve their athletic performance. The path to muscle building and athletic prowess, on the other hand, is subtle and frequently overlooked by weight loss tactics. Carbohydrate cycling, while popular for weight loss, is a great but underutilized technique for body contouring and athletic performance.

Muscle hypertrophy requires a complex mix of nutrition, resistance training, and rest, with carbohydrates playing an important role. Carbohydrates are the body's major energy source, powering strenuous exercises and stimulating muscle recovery and growth. Muscles develop small tears after an intensive workout, which, when mended through protein synthesis, result in muscular growth. Carbohydrates supply the energy required for this repair process by delivering amino acids into the muscles, so promoting recovery and growth.

Carb-cycling's rhythmic alternation of high and low-carb days corresponds nicely with a muscle-building diet. On hard training days, high-carb days replenish glycogen levels, facilitating recuperation and preparation for the next workout, whereas low-carb days on rest or low-intensity days enable effective fat utilization and lean muscle maintenance.

Athletic performance, while related to muscle growth, has different energy requirements depending on the intensity and length of the exercise. Carbohydrate cycling can be customized to satisfy these requirements, guaranteeing adequate glycogen levels for high-intensity activities and efficient fat utilization for endurance activities. Carbohydrates also have an impact on hormone levels, particularly cortisol and insulin. Carbohydrates can lower post-workout cortisol levels, promoting a muscle-building environment, and regulate insulin to improve nutrition uptake by muscles, aiding in recuperation and growth.

Individual carbohydrate sensitivities, training routines, and recuperation requirements differ, making it critical to listen to one's body and adjust carb-cycling properly. It is a path of refining and adaptation.

Carb-Cycling for Special Populations (Vegans, Seniors, etc.)

Dietary regimens, while universal in their fundamental concepts, frequently require customisation. This is especially true when we consider humanity's various tapestry, each with their own set of requirements, interests, and life stages. Carb-cycling, a flexible and adjustable method, is no exception. While its essential concepts stay similar, how it is executed varies, particularly for unique populations such as vegans, elders, and others.

Let's start with a voyage across the vegan world. Vegans, whether by choice or need, avoid all animal products. While this lifestyle is ethical and environmentally responsible, it poses unique dietary issues, especially when combined with carb-cycling. What is the key concern? Sources of protein. While carb-cycling stresses the cyclical consumption of carbohydrates, protein is a continuous companion that is essential for muscle repair and satisfaction. Traditional protein sources such as meat, dairy, and eggs are not acceptable to vegans. Instead, they rely on plant-based substitutes like as lentils, beans, tofu, and tempeh. When planning a carb-cycling menu for vegans, it's critical to include these protein sources, especially on low-carb days. Furthermore, many grains and legumes, which are staples in a vegan diet, are high in carbohydrates. Striking a balance, guaranteeing appropriate protein without exceeding carb limitations, becomes an art.

Let us now turn our attention to our elderly, a generation that is often disregarded in the fitness world but is equally deserving of health and vitality. Our metabolic rate and muscle mass naturally fall as we age. Carbohydrate cycling for seniors then serves a dual purpose: it preserves lean muscle while controlling energy intake to avoid undesirable weight gain. The approach here is cautious, ensuring that any carbohydrate reduction does not result in weariness or nutrient shortages. Furthermore, bone health takes precedence, thus foods high in calcium and vitamin D, regardless of carb level, should be preferred.

Other unique demographics, such as pregnant women or people with certain medical concerns, will necessitate even more customized approaches, always under the supervision of healthcare specialists. The beauty of carb-cycling is its adaptability. It is a flexible framework that bends and adapts to meet the specific needs of each individual.

While carb-cycling provides a road map, it is up to each individual to chart their own path based on their particular life circumstances. Carb-cycling may be molded, shaped, and adjusted to meet your individual health needs, whether you're a vegan athlete, a senior trying to preserve vitality, or someone with specific health issues.

Chapter 8: Synergizing Carb-Cycling with Workouts

Carb-cycling is more than just a change in diet; it's a complex tango between eating well and working exercise. Carb-cycling and exercise have a remarkable synergy that we'll discuss in Chapter 8. This section provides an in-depth approach to making the most of carb-cycling through strategic exercise, from learning the science underlying exercise and carb utilization to developing workout regimens that are specific to high-carb and low-carb days. As we progress, we'll also discuss the often-overlooked but critically important factors of recuperation and rest, highlighting their significance in this all-encompassing strategy for health and fitness.

The Science of Exercise and Carb Utilization

Few issues are as linked in the huge world of fitness and nutrition as exercise and carbohydrate usage. To really understand the synergy between them, one must first go deep into the molecular ballet that unfolds within our muscles during physical activity. This complicated and dynamic dance is powered primarily by carbs, the body's primary source of rapid energy. But how precisely does this process function, and what role does carb-cycling play in enhancing our workouts? Let us go on this fascinating adventure together.

Consider yourself about to begin a high-intensity workout. Your pulse rate quickens in anticipation, and your muscles tense up as you take that initial step, jump, or lift. These muscles, like a car, require fuel. This is when carbohydrates come into play. These carbs, which are stored in our muscles and liver as glycogen, are quickly broken down into glucose, which then enters the powerhouse of our cells, the mitochondria, to produce energy.

Now, the type of exercise you do has a big impact on how your body uses these carbs. Aerobic workouts, such as long-distance running or swimming, rely on a combination of carbs and lipids for energy. However, as the intensity of the exercise increases, the dependency on carbs becomes more obvious. Why? Simply put, carbs give more energy than fats, making them important for brief, strong spurts of exercise.

Conversely, during low-intensity exercises or rest times, the body relies more on fat reserves for energy, protecting those valuable glycogen stores. This subtle alteration in glucose and fat utilization demonstrates the body's extraordinary adaptability.

Enter carb-cycling. When combined with exercise, this nutritional strategy, with its rhythmic adjustment of glucose intake, can be a game changer. On high-carb days, which should ideally coincide with high-intensity workouts, regenerated glycogen stores guarantee that muscles have enough fuel to operate properly. The increase in dietary carbs also causes an increase in insulin, a hormone that, in addition to regulating blood sugar, is important in transporting nutrients into cells, which aids post-workout recovery.

On the other hand, on low-carb days, which may coincide with rest days or low-intensity workouts, the body gets more adept at dipping into fat reserves for energy. This not only aids in fat loss but also trains the body to become metabolically flexible, smoothly switching between different energy sources.

While the physics behind exercise and glucose utilization is fascinating, it's important to note that everyone's response is different. Genetics, fitness levels, and even the time of day can all influence how the body processes and utilises carbs during exercise. For example, some people may discover that they have better stamina for morning workouts on high-carb days, while others may find that they perform best in the evenings.

Furthermore, hydration and electrolyte balance, which are frequently disregarded, play an important role in optimizing glucose utilization during exercise. Carbohydrates drive water into cells, and appropriate fluid intake can have a substantial impact on muscular function and recovery.

The tango between exercise and carbohydrates is a delicate balance, a duet that involves insight, intuition, and occasionally a bit of trial and error. However, using carb-cycling as a guiding framework, one may harness the power of carbs not just as a nutritional component, but as a strategic tool, boosting workouts, accelerating recovery, and propelling one towards their fitness goals.

Understanding the science of exercise and glucose utilization can be motivating in the fitness world, where misconceptions frequently obscure reality. It demystifies the method, allowing users to make informed decisions, adjust their routines, and truly make the most of their carb-cycling experience. After all, knowledge, when employed, is power. And in this situation, it's the ability to transform, invigorate, and thrive.

Workout Plans for High-Carb and Low-Carb Days

Starting a carb-cycling adventure is about more than just the food on your plate. It's a comprehensive method that combines nutrition and exercise, with each complimenting the other in a dance of energy, recovery, and results. Understanding how to match workouts to high-carb and low-carb days can be the key to realizing the full potential of this nutritional strategy for novices. Let's go into the specifics of creating the best training regimens for these specific days.

Your body is like a car with a full tank of gas on high-carb days. Your muscles' increased glycogen stores are begging to be spent, making now an excellent time to indulge in high-intensity workouts. Consider activities that get your heart pumping, your sweat dripping, and your muscles burning. These workouts are often shorter in time but high in intensity.

Workouts for a High-Carb Day:

Alternate running and walking for cardio intervals. Sprint for 30 seconds, then walk or jog for one minute. This not only increases your metabolism but also takes use of the available energy from carbs.

Strength Training: With plenty of energy available, this is an excellent day to tackle greater muscle groups. Squats, deadlifts, and bench presses are examples of compound motions. These exercises work numerous muscles at the same time, resulting in a larger calorie burn.

Circuit training is quickly transitioning from one activity to the next while keeping the heart rate elevated. A circuit could comprise a combination of aerobic, strength, and plyometric movements to provide a full-body workout.

Low-carb days, on the other hand, are when the body's glycogen reserves are depleted. While doing out on certain days may seem paradoxical, the body's improved ability to dip into fat reserves for energy can be exploited with the correct kind of activities.

Workouts for a Low-Carb Day:

Steady-State Cardio: Instead of short bursts of high-intensity cardio, opt for extended periods of moderate-intensity cardio. Exercises such as brisk walking, cycling, or swimming are great. They enable the body to use fat as its primary fuel source without exhausting its already depleted glycogen stores.

Yoga and Pilates are great for low-carb days. They emphasize flexibility, balance, and core strength, allowing a reprieve from the high-intensity workouts of high-carb days while still providing a plethora of advantages.

Resistance Training: Focus on isolation exercises that target specific muscles with lighter weights and higher repetitions. Consider tricep extensions, bicep curls, and leg curls. The goal is to engage the muscles while not overworking the body.

Let's turn this knowledge into a concrete workout regimen for beginners:

Table: Carb-Cycling Workout Plan for Beginners

Day Type	Workout	Duration	Intensity
High-Carb	Cardio Intervals	20 minutes	High
	Strength Training (Squats, Deadlifts)	30 minutes	Moderate to High
	Circuit Training (Jumping Jacks, Push-ups, Lunges)	25 minutes	High
Low-Carb	Brisk Walking	40 minutes	Moderate
	Yoga	30 minutes	Low to Moderate
	Resistance Training (Bicep Curls, Leg Curls)	25 minutes	Moderate

Incorporating these workouts into your carb-cycling routine can be transformative. However, it's essential to listen to your body. Some days, you might feel like pushing harder, while on others, a gentle yoga session might be all you can muster. And that's okay. The journey of fitness and health is deeply personal, and while guidelines can point you in the right direction, your body's signals are the ultimate guide. Embrace the process, enjoy the workouts, and watch as carb-cycling and exercise synergize to propel you towards your goals.

Recovery, Rest Days, and Carb-Cycling

Recovery is an often-overlooked component of fitness and nutrition that plays a critical part in our quest for maximum health. While the adrenaline rush of a hard workout or the joy of a well-executed high-carb day might be intoxicating, it's the quiet times of rest and recuperation that truly determine our growth. We'll discover the significant impact of these aspects on our general well-being as we delve into the intricate relationship between recuperation, rest days, and carb-cycling.

Consider our bodies to be complicated bits of equipment for a moment. Just as a car need regular maintenance and occasional downtime to perform well, our bodies require rest periods to heal, regenerate, and thrive. This is especially true when we incorporate a dynamic program like carb-cycling into our lives.

Rest days may appear to be unhelpful on the surface. After all, aren't we supposed to be moving, pushing, and challenging ourselves all the time? However, it is during these periods of rest that our muscles repair the micro-tears created by rigorous training, resulting in enhanced growth and strength. Furthermore, our bodies are skilled at utilizing these opportunities to regulate hormones, refill glycogen stores, and reduce inflammation.

Let's now add carb-cycling to the equation. Our bodies are inundated with the necessary fuel to support these activities on high-carb days, when our exercises are more intense. But what about low-carb days, which frequently coincide with relaxation or light exercise? These days, we may help our bodies recuperate by allowing them to use fat stores for energy, promoting hormonal balance, and easing the load on our digestive systems.

Strategically placing carbs around workouts can improve recuperation. Consuming carbohydrates post-workout can hasten glycogen regeneration, allowing for faster recovery and minimizing muscular discomfort. This connection between carb intake and recovery demonstrates the all-encompassing nature of carb-cycling.

Chapter 9: Real-Life Journeys: Success Stories and Lessons

Carb-cycling is like a fingerprint; everyone's experience with it is different. Even if the underlying science and concepts are the same for everyone, the specific struggles, triumphs, and lessons are what make each person's journey unique. Chapter 9 dives into these anecdotes, weaving together a tapestry of events ranging from the profoundly life-altering to the merely insightful. These accounts aren't just about becoming in shape, but rather about finding one's true identity, strengthening one's resolve, and developing a more meaningful connection to one's body and well-being. We are reminded as we move through these stories that the human spirit, with its resiliency and flexibility, is the true engine of change, not carb-cycling.

Personal Narratives of Transformation

Personal stories have a particular force in the huge terrain of health and fitness. They're more than just triumphant stories or failed lessons; they're personal experiences that resonate, motivate, and reflect our own goals. As we go deeper into the world of carb-cycling, it is these transformational stories that truly bring the science, methods, and schedules to life. We get insights from individuals who have walked the route that no textbook or guide can provide.

Consider the case of Elena, a 35-year-old mother of two. Elena felt that her post-pregnancy weight was an immovable shadow. She'd tried every diet in the book, from juice cleanses to raw food diets, but her weight hadn't budged. But it wasn't just about the weight. The endless cycle of dieting left her psychologically and physically exhausted. Then she discovered carb-cycling. The notion piqued her interest not because it promised weight loss, but because it took a holistic approach to health. Elena started her journey by alternating between high and low carb days. Within months, she noticed not just a large weight loss, but also an increase in energy, more stable moods, and a transformation in her relationship with food. Elena saw carb-cycling as more than simply a diet; it was a way of life.

Then there's Jamal, a collegiate athlete who was always in great form. However, a knee injury suffered during a game forced him to miss months of recuperation and inactivity. Jamal's confidence fell as he saw his hard-earned muscles deteriorate and his weight rise. He understood he needed a strategy to help him restore his lost shape and increase his performance when he was finally cleared to workout again. That's when he discovered carb-cycling. Jamal followed a well planned diet that included high-carb days to fuel his intensive exercises and low-carb days to maximize fat burn. The outcome was nothing short of astounding. He not only regained his athletic form, but he also set personal records in his performance measures.

While Elena and Jamal's tales are very different, they are linked by a common thread: the transforming impact of carb-cycling. However, keep in mind that each path is unique. For some, the transition may be sudden and spectacular, while for others, it may be gradual and continuous. Then there's Priya, a vegan who struggled at first to incorporate carb-cycling into her plant-based diet. But, with a little research, imagination, and patience, she devised a vegan carb-cycling regimen that not only coincided with her ethical principles but also provided amazing health advantages.

These diverse stories highlight a key truth about carb-cycling: it is not a one-size-fits-all method. It's adaptive, elastic, and very personal. As we read these stories, we're reminded that every transformation is the result of a journey filled with struggles, wins, lessons, and moments of introspection. And, while carb-cycling science offers the framework, it is the human spirit, with its unbreakable will and tenacity, that actually brings it to life.

Finally, these personal stories offer as evidence of carb-cycling's transformational power. They provide hope, motivation, and a road map for individuals at a crossroads, asking if this is the correct path for them. We are reminded, via the lived experiences of Elena, Jamal, Priya, and countless others, that transformation is more than just exterior appearances; it is an inner journey of rediscovery.

Overcoming Challenges: Tips from Those Who've Been There

Every voyage, no matter how well-planned, will have rocky parts. The carb-cycling path, however transformative, is not an exception. As we traverse the complexities of this dietary strategy, we will undoubtedly confront challenges—some expected, others unanticipated. But, as the old saying goes, it is not the obstacles we face that define us, but how we respond to them. And who better to lead us through these trials than people who have walked the journey, stumbled, pulled themselves up, and come out stronger?

Consider Rosa, a diligent professional juggling the responsibilities of a demanding job and a busy family life. The problem for Rosa was not comprehending the principles of carb-cycling or even incorporating them into her everyday routine. Instead, it was social occasions like meals, parties, and gatherings that were difficult. How can one keep to a carb-cycling strategy while surrounded by tempting foods? Rosa's solution was simple but brilliant. She started hosting potluck meals, where she prepared a carb-cycling-friendly main dish and visitors brought sides. This way, she assured that there were always options that fit her diet, and she introduced her friends to the delectable versatility of carb-cycling dishes.

Alex is a college student living in a dorm with limited kitchen amenities. The challenge for him was to create carb-cycling meals using only a microwave and a mini-fridge. Alex resorted to no-cook dishes, overnight oats, salads, and wraps. He also purchased a tiny blender, which allows him to make protein-packed smoothies on his low-carb days. His path emphasizes the significance of adaptation and the idea that any problem can be overcome with a little inventiveness.

Many people, including Lila, had an internal problem. The initial excitement of starting carb-cycling was evident, but motivation dwindled as the days moved into weeks. Many of us may identify with the initial surge of inspiration that gradually fades. What is Lila's solution? She began a notebook in which she recorded not just her meals but also her feelings, struggles, and achievements. On days when she wasn't feeling motivated, she'd go back through her entries, drawing strength from her previous accomplishments and utilizing her disappointments as lessons.

These stories, full of grit and resourcefulness, provide essential lessons. They serve as a reminder that, while difficult, obstacles are not insurmountable. Any problem may be turned into an opportunity with determination, imagination, and a dash of ingenuity. And as we embark on our carb-cycling adventure, armed with the wisdom of those who have gone before us, we are not only better prepared to meet problems; we are also ready to turn them into stepping stones to success.

Chapter 10: Troubleshooting and Common Concerns

No matter how meticulously one plans a trip, there are bound to be unforeseen detours along the way. Carb-cycling's route is similarly revolutionary but not unique. In Chapter 10, we look into the most frequent worries and difficulties encountered along the way. We will investigate all sorts of obstacles, from those that put our body to the test to those that test our mental fortitude. With the right information, perspective, and plan of action, you can overcome these obstacles and have a productive and illuminating carb-cycling experience.

Addressing Dietary Challenges: Cost, Time, and Ingredients

Setting off on a carb-cycling adventure is like to setting sail on unexplored waters. The promise of transformative beaches beckons, but the journey is not without its difficulties. The perceived expenses, time effort, and availability of specific products are among the most prominent concerns for individuals new to this nutritional strategy. Let us go into these issues in depth, refuting myths and providing real solutions for each.

Cost: There is a widespread belief that eating healthily or adhering to a specific dietary plan is expensive. It's easy to be misled by the attraction of processed meals, which are frequently less expensive and more easily available. But the truth is that carb-cycling does not have to be expensive. It is all about making informed decisions. Buying in bulk, for example, can often result in large savings. Grains, seeds, and certain non-perishable goods can be stored for extended periods of time, and the cost per serving is frequently lower when purchased in bulk.

Farmers' markets may be treasure troves of fresh, local products, frequently at lower rates than supermarkets. Engaging with local farmers can also provide insights into seasonal produce, which is often less expensive and more fresh. Consider purchasing a membership to a wholesale club as well. The initial purchase may appear high, but the long-term savings on pantry goods can be significant.

Time: "I just don't have the time!" It's a song we've all heard, if not said ourselves. Making time for meal preparation can be difficult with work, family, and the many demands of modern life. But here's a surprise: with a little planning, carb-cycling can be easily integrated into even the busiest of schedules.

Weekends and off days can be used to prepare meals for the coming week. Consider the ease of reaching into your fridge and finding a carb-friendly meal ready to go. It's about assuring consistency in your carb-cycling path, not just convenience. Remember, not every meal has to be a gourmet occasion. Simple, nutritious meals are frequently the most appealing to our taste buds and nutritional goals.

Consider batch cooking on days when even the concept of cooking is daunting. This method of cooking in bulk and freezing portions ensures that you always have a meal ready to go. It's not only a time saving; on very frantic days, it's a lifeline.

Ingredients: "I can't find that specific ingredient!" Whether it's a specific grain, a seed, or a unique vegetable, the carb-cycling trip can feel like a scavenger hunt at times. But here's the thing: carb-cycling is really adaptable. Can't seem to find quinoa? Make use of millet. Are you missing chia seeds? Flaxseeds are a great replacement. Understanding the basic ideas and adapting them to what's available is the heart of carb-cycling, not simply following to a set ingredient list.

Moreover, in our digitally connected age, numerous online retailers specialize in delivering even the most obscure ingredients right to your doorstep. However, before you click the 'purchase' button, examine whether there is a local alternative. This not only helps local businesses, but it also lowers the carbon footprint of your meals.

Carb-cycling, like any worthwhile pursuit, needs dedication, a little ingenuity, and a willingness to adapt. But the benefits—a healthier body, a better understanding of nutrition, and the sheer pleasure of eating tasty, nutritious meals—are well worth the effort. And remember that every struggle you confront and overcome is not only a testimonial to your tenacity, but also a step closer to your transformational goals.

Social and Lifestyle Challenges: Dining Out, Social Events, and Travel

Starting a carb-cycling journey is more than simply a personal challenge; it's a lifestyle adjustment that affects every aspect of our lives. While the kitchen is the beginning point, the trip goes far beyond its walls. For someone trying to navigate the carb-cycling route, the real world, with its various social engagements, dining out experiences, and vacation adventures, may sometimes feel like a maze. Let us investigate these difficulties and equip ourselves with solutions to meet them front on.

Dining Out: The ambiance of a restaurant, the aroma of dishes wafting from the kitchen, the chatter of patrons—dining out is an experience, a break from routine. But for someone on a carb-cycling diet, it can also be a minefield. Menus don't always cater to specific dietary needs, and the fear of deviating from one's carb-cycling plan can cast a shadow over the entire experience.

However, with a bit of foresight, dining out can be a delightful experience, even on this diet. Start by researching the restaurant's menu online. Many establishments now offer detailed nutritional information, allowing you to plan your meal ahead of time. If the menu seems restrictive, don't hesitate to communicate with the staff. Chefs often appreciate the challenge of catering to specific dietary needs and might surprise you with a delicious, carb-appropriate dish.

Another strategy is to time your dining out experiences with your high-carb days, giving you a broader range of options. But remember, it's not just about the carbs; it's about making wholesome choices. Opt for grilled over fried, choose dishes rich in vegetables, and be mindful of portion sizes.

Social Events: From birthdays to weddings, social events are a celebration of life's milestones. They're also a veritable buffet of dietary challenges. Cakes, pastries, cocktails—temptations abound. The key to navigating social events is balance. If you know you'll be attending an event, plan your meals around it. Maybe it's a high-carb day, allowing you a bit more flexibility. Or perhaps you choose to indulge a little but balance it out with a more rigorous workout.

It's also essential to remember that social events are about more than just food. They're about connections, laughter, shared memories. Focus on the people, the conversations, the joy of the moment. Food is just one part of the equation.

Travel: Ah, the allure of new destinations, the thrill of exploration! But travel also means a break from routine, from the comfort of your kitchen and your meal prep. The key to carb-cycling while traveling is preparation. If you're flying, consider packing a meal or snacks. Many airlines offer specific meal requests, but having your own ensures you stay on track.

When dining out, embrace local cuisine but make informed choices. Opt for dishes that align with your carb-cycling plan. And remember, travel is also an opportunity for physical activity. Explore on foot, go for a swim, or even try a local sport or activity.

Dining out becomes an opportunity to advocate for your needs, social events transform into celebrations of more than just food, and travel? Well, it's a chance to take your carb-cycling journey global. Every challenge faced is a lesson learned, a testament to your commitment, and a step closer to your transformational goals.

Physical and Mental Challenges: Energy Slumps, Cravings, and Mindset

Setting off on a carb-cycling adventure is like to setting sail on unexplored waters. The prospect of new horizons is exciting, but the journey is not without its challenges. The physical and mental tempests that anchor us down, the cravings that threaten to steer us off course, and the mindset that may either be our compass or our downfall are among the most daunting hurdles that people sailing this nutritional sea encounter.

Energy Slumps: It's a feeling that many of us have experienced. You might be full of vigor, ready to tackle the world, and then you can be exhausted, battling to keep your eyes open. Energy slumps are a normal component of our bodies' rhythms, but while carb-cycling, these dips might feel more pronounced. Because the body is acclimated to a certain fuel intake, it may initially fight the adjustments, resulting in fatigue. But there is a silver lining: these downturns are only brief. Energy levels stabilize as the body adjusts to the new routine. To avoid these dips, make sure you're getting enough fats and proteins on low-carb days. These macronutrients can serve as alternate energy sources, keeping you afloat.

Cravings: Oh, the allure of forbidden foods! Just as sailors were tempted to the enticing melodies of sirens, we can be drawn to the appeal of off-plan foods. Cravings aren't only bodily; they're also strongly linked to our emotions and memories. Combating them necessitates a two-pronged strategy. Physically, eat nutrient-dense foods to keep yourself full. Cravings are less likely to occur when one's stomach is full. Investigate the source of the craving mentally. Is it a longing for a childhood treat? Or is it tension that seeks consolation in comfort food? Recognizing emotional triggers allows us to address the underlying issue instead of succumbing to the need.

Mindset: The commander of our carb-cycling ship is our mentality. Doubts and negativity can sink our efforts, whereas a positive, resilient mindset can weather any storm. It is critical to cultivate a development mindset, one that views setbacks as chances for growth rather than insurmountable hurdles. Surround yourself with positive people, whether through online communities or local support groups. Celebrate the tiny triumphs, and remember that every setback serves as a springboard for a return.

Chapter 11: Advanced Carb-Cycling Strategies

Carb-cycling is a dietary method that has recently acquired popularity due to its potential benefits in optimizing body composition, boosting athletic performance, and maintaining general health. To regulate carbohydrate consumption and maximize the body's metabolic response, this strategy entails alternating between high-carb and low-carb days. While carbohydrate cycling can be beneficial for many people, it is not a one-size-fits-all strategy. This chapter will go into greater detail on advanced carb-cycling tactics that can be adapted to your specific requirements and goals. We'll look at the relationship between intermittent fasting and carb-cycling, the possibility of combining carb-cycling with ketosis, and how to modify carb-cycling for different forms of exercise. Understanding these advanced tactics will allow you to customize your carb-cycling diet to your specific needs and maximize your outcomes.

Intermittent Fasting and Carb-Cycling Synergy

As you learn more about carb-cycling, you may come across another nutritional method that has been making headlines in the health and fitness community: intermittent fasting. These two approaches may appear to be diametrically opposed at first glance. Carb-cycling involves varying carbohydrate consumption throughout the week, whereas intermittent fasting entails alternating between eating and fasting times. When you look closely, you'll notice that these two tactics can really compliment one other in a lovely synergistic dance.

Intermittent fasting is about when you eat rather than what you eat. The most frequent method entails fasting for a set number of hours each day, usually between 16 and 20, and then eating all of your meals within a set time frame, usually 4 to 8 hours. This eating and fasting routine helps to control insulin levels, increase fat reduction, and stimulate autophagy, the body's natural cellular cleansing mechanism.

Carb-cycling, on the other hand, is all about what you eat. It entails alternating between high-carb days, during which you consume more carbohydrates to fuel your workouts and replenish glycogen levels, and low-carb days, during which you limit your carb intake to urge your body to use fat stores for energy.

Let us now discuss the synergy. When you mix intermittent fasting and carb-cycling, you create a potent combo that can boost metabolic function, fat loss, and general health. Your body is already programmed to use fat as fuel on low-carb days. By integrating intermittent fasting on certain days, you can increase fat burning by increasing the time your body is fasted. On high-carb days, on the other hand, you can time your carb consumption around your exercises and within your eating window to maximize glycogen replenishment and muscle repair.

It's worth noting that, while this combo can be extremely powerful, it's not for everyone. It necessitates some metabolic flexibility as well as an understanding of your individual body's requirements and responses. Before making any significant changes to your diet or exercise program, always consult with a healthcare provider or a licensed nutritionist.

Carb-Cycling in Ketosis: Is It Possible?

One of the most commonly asked questions by individuals new to carb-cycling and ketogenic eating is if the two can be combined. It may appear conflicting at first. The ketogenic diet is a low-carb, high-fat diet that tries to keep your body in ketosis, a state in which it burns fat for fuel rather than carbs. Carb-cycling, on the other hand, includes rotating between high-carb and low-carb days, which appears to contradict ketosis principles. However, with little forethought and an awareness of how your body reacts to different macronutrients, it is possible to combine carb-cycling and ketosis in a way that optimizes your outcomes.

Let's start by delving deeper into the science of ketosis. When you eat carbs, your body transforms them into glucose, which is subsequently used to generate energy. Any surplus glucose is stored as glycogen in your muscles and liver, and if those stores are depleted, it is stored as fat. When your carbohydrate consumption is dramatically reduced, as in the ketogenic diet, your body depletes its glycogen stores and begins to break down fat into ketones, which can be used for energy. This is referred to as ketosis.

Let's talk about carb-cycling now. Carb-cycling is the practice of adjusting your carbohydrate intake to maximize your body's metabolic reaction. You consume extra carbohydrates on high-carb days to restore glycogen stores and fuel your exercises. You limit your carbohydrate consumption on low-carb days to urge your body to use its fat stores for energy. This method is especially advantageous for those who engage in regular, intensive exercise because it allows for optimal performance and recovery while also encouraging fat loss.

So, how do you mix carbohydrate cycling with ketosis? The idea is to plan out your carbohydrate consumption. On low-carb days, you can adopt a ketogenic diet, consuming very little carbohydrates, moderate protein, and a lot of fat. This will induce ketosis in your body and cause it to burn fat for fuel. You can boost your carbohydrate consumption on high-carb days, but you must do so strategically. Consume high-quality, complex carbs such as sweet potatoes, quinoa, and whole grains, and plan your meals around your workouts. This will help your body to refill glycogen stores and enhance muscle repair without knocking you out of ketosis for a long time.

It is vital to note that moving into and out of ketosis does not happen instantaneously. It can take your body several hours to many days to go from burning glucose to burning ketones, and vice versa. As a result, it's critical to pay attention to how your body reacts to dietary changes and adjust accordingly. For example, if you feel sluggish and short on energy following a high-carb day, reducing your carbohydrate consumption or increasing the duration of your low-carb days may be beneficial.

Furthermore, keep in mind that everyone's body is unique, and what works for one person may not work for another. Before making any significant changes to your diet or exercise program, always consult with a healthcare provider or a licensed nutritionist.

You can reap the benefits of both techniques by being selective about your carbohydrate consumption and paying attention to how your body responds. Before making any significant changes to your food or exercise program, talk with a healthcare provider or a qualified nutritionist, and always listen to your body.

Adapting Carb-Cycling for Endurance vs. Strength Training.

Carbohydrate cycling is a dietary strategy that involves alternating between high-carb and low-carb days. This strategy optimizes carbohydrate consumption for energy, muscle building, and fat removal. However, the type of training you do, whether endurance or strength training, can have a huge impact on how you build your carb-cycling regimen. Both types of training have different energy demands and so necessitate a different carb-cycling strategy.

Training for Endurance

Endurance training entails long durations of moderate-intensity activity, such as jogging, cycling, or swimming. This style of exercise is primarily based on aerobic metabolism, which uses carbs and fats as key energy sources. During endurance activity, your body will initially use glycogen as a source of energy, which is the stored form of carbs in your muscles and liver. As glycogen levels dwindle, your body will become more reliant on fat for energy. Carbohydrates, on the other hand, are still necessary for peak performance since they are a more efficient source of energy than lipids.

It is critical for endurance athletes to have adequate glycogen stored in their muscles and liver to maintain energy levels during their workout. As a result, it is helpful to consume more carbohydrates in the days preceding and following a lengthy endurance activity. This will restore your glycogen stores and provide you with enough energy to perform at your peak. Reduce your carbohydrate consumption on rest days or days when you are doing light exercise to encourage your body to utilise fat as a source of energy.

Strengthening Exercises

Weightlifting, bodyweight exercises, and high-intensity interval training (HIIT) are examples of workouts that need short bursts of energy at a high intensity. This style of exercise is primarily based on anaerobic metabolism, which employs carbohydrates as the primary energy source. Your body will use glycogen as a source of energy during strength training, and it is critical to have enough glycogen stored in your muscles to function at your best.

It is helpful to have a greater carbohydrate intake on days when you are conducting your most strenuous exercises if you are undertaking strength training. This will restore your glycogen stores and provide you with enough energy to perform at your peak. Reduce your carbohydrate consumption on rest days or days when you are doing light exercise to encourage your body to utilise fat as a source of energy.

Carbohydrate Cycling for Training

It is critical to consider the intensity and duration of your workouts while modifying carb-cycling for training. A larger carbohydrate intake is useful on days when you are conducting intensive or prolonged exercise to replenish glycogen stores and maximize performance. Reduce your carbohydrate consumption on rest days or days when you are doing light exercise to encourage your body to utilise fat as a source of energy.

It is also critical to examine the time of your carbohydrate consumption. Consuming carbohydrates before your workout will help you perform better, while carbohydrates after your workout can help you replace glycogen stores and recover faster.

The key to successfully adapting carb-cycling for your training is to listen to your body and observe how it reacts to various levels of carbohydrate consumption. It may take some time and experimentation to find the perfect technique for you, but with patience and perseverance, you can optimize your carb-cycling diet to complement your training goals.

Chapter 12: 4-Week Carb-Cycling Meal Plan

Week 1: Introduction and Getting Started

Starting a new diet may be both exhilarating and intimidating. As your body and mind acclimate to a new way of eating and living, the first week is generally the most difficult. However, with the appropriate mindset and preparation, you may position yourself for success right away. The carb cycling diet is a versatile and successful method for weight loss and overall wellness. To improve your body's metabolism and fat-burning capacities, alternate between high-carb, low-carb, and no-carb days. As a beginner, you must begin cautiously and progressively increase your understanding and practice of carb cycling.

The first week of your carb cycling adventure is all about getting started and building the groundwork for the weeks ahead. This week must be approached with an open mind and a cheerful attitude. Remember that it is normal to make mistakes and face difficulties along the path. The trick is to learn from them while remaining focused on your objectives.

Begin by defining specific and attainable goals for yourself. Having a clear picture of what you want to achieve will help keep you motivated and focused, whether you want to reduce weight, grow muscle, or improve your athletic performance. Next, become acquainted with the fundamentals of carb cycling. Understanding the concepts of carb cycling and how it works can allow you to make more informed diet and activity decisions.

Any diet requires planning to be successful, and carb cycling is no exception. Spend some time planning your weekly meals and exercise program. Consider your schedule as well as any social or professional obligations you may have. Finding a balance that works for you and fits into your lifestyle is critical. Remember that carb cycling is a flexible method that allows for modifications as needed.

It is critical to focus on entire, nutrient-dense foods throughout the first week. Include a wide range of lean proteins, healthy fats, and carbohydrates in your diet. On high-carb days, prioritize complex carbs such as whole grains, legumes, and starchy vegetables. Prioritize lean proteins and healthy fats on low-carb days, and limit carbohydrate intake to non-starchy veggies. On no-carb days, focus on lean proteins and healthy fats while avoiding carbohydrates entirely.

Exercise is an essential part of the carb cycling diet. On high-carb days, moderate to intense exercise is advised, whereas light to moderate exercise is advised on low-carb and no-carb days. However, it is critical to listen to your body and make any adjustments to your exercise regimen. If you are new to exercise or have not been active in a long time, it is critical to begin carefully and gradually build your intensity and length.

The first week of any new diet can be difficult, and it is normal to have ups and downs. Keep a positive attitude, be motivated, and remember why you began this path in the first place. You can set yourself up for success and establish a solid foundation for the weeks ahead if you have the correct mindset and preparation.

Day	Breakfast	Lunch	Snack	Dinner
1	Banana Berry Oatmeal	Chickpea and Vegetable Stir-Fry	Apple and Almond Butter Sandwich or Baked Apple with Cinnamon	Spaghetti Squash with Tomato Sauce and Parmesan
2	Whole Grain Pancakes with Apple and Nuts	Quinoa and Black Bean Salad	Berry and Banana Smoothie or Chocolate and Banana Mug Cake	Lentil and Vegetable Stuffed Bell Peppers
3	Quinoa and	Sweet Potato and	Peanut Butter and Jelly Energy	Sweet Potato and

Day	Breakfast	Lunch	Snack	Dinner
	Vegetable Breakfast Bowl	Lentil Curry	Bites or Berry and Yogurt Parfait	Chickpea Curry
4	Scrambled Eggs with Spinach and Feta	Grilled Chicken Salad	Chocolate and Banana Smoothie or Oatmeal and Peanut Butter Cookies	Zucchini Noodles with Pesto and Cherry Tomatoes
5	Almond Flour Pancakes	Shrimp and Avocado Salad	Trail Mix or Pineapple and Coconut Sorbet	Lemon Garlic Roasted Chicken
6	Chia Seed Pudding	Beef and Broccoli Stir-Fry	Fruit and Nut Bars or Chocolate and Avocado Mousse	Baked Salmon with Asparagus
7	Flaxseed Muffins	Turkey and Cheese Lettuce Wraps	Oatmeal and Raisin Energy Bites or Apple and Cinnamon Muffins	Beef Stir-Fry with Broccoli

Week 2: Refining and Adjusting Based on Feedback

As you enter the second week of your carb-cycling journey, it's time to assess your progress and make any required adjustments. The first week was spent setting the tone and settling into the new routine. Now is the time to pay attention to your body and see how it reacts to the changes. Do you have more energy now? Have your weight or body composition changed recently? Are there any meals or exercises that you really like or dislike?

It's critical to realize that carb cycling isn't a one-size-fits-all solution. It's a versatile diet plan that may be adapted to your own needs and interests. So, if necessary, make adjustments to your meal plan or workout schedule. Consider boosting your carb intake somewhat if you find yourself feeling exhausted on low-carb days. Alternatively, if you feel that particular workouts are too tough for you, adapt them to a more comfortable level.

It is also critical to pay attention to your mental and emotional well-being. Carb cycling can be mentally taxing, especially at first. It is reasonable to feel doubt or dissatisfaction. However, it is critical to remain optimistic and devoted to the process. Remember that it is acceptable to take days off. What matters is how you recover and stay on track.

Don't forget to enjoy the tiny victories. Take time to notice and celebrate your achievement, whether it's sticking to your eating plan, completing a difficult workout, or simply feeling good in your body. These modest triumphs will motivate you and urge you onward on your carb-cycling path.

Day	Breakfast	Lunch	Snack	Dinner
8	Sweet Potato and Black Bean Hash	Vegetable and Bean Burrito	Cucumber and Hummus Roll-Ups or Berry Protein Gelato	Vegetable and Bean Pasta
9	Peanut Butter and Banana Smoothie	Lentil and Vegetable Stew	Almond and Coconut Energy Bites or Protein Chocolate Pudding	Quinoa and Vegetable Stir-Fry
10	Apple and Cinnamon Porridge	Vegetable and Quinoa Stir-Fry	Avocado and Tomato Salsa or Protein Cheesecake Bites	Chickpea and Tomato Stew
11	Coconut Flour Waffles	Chicken and Vegetable	Berry and Chia Seed Pudding or Protein Chocolate Chip Cookies	Pork Chops with Green Beans

Day	Breakfast	Lunch	Snack	Dinner
		Skewers		
12	Smoked Salmon and Cream Cheese Omelette	Tuna Salad Stuffed Avocado	Cheese and Vegetable Sticks or Protein Lemon Bars	Shrimp Scampi with Zucchini Noodles
13	Almond and Berry Smoothie	Egg Salad Lettuce Wraps	Chocolate and Almond Smoothie or Protein-Packed Peanut Butter Cups	Grilled Steak with Roasted Vegetables
14	Avocado and Tomato Salad	Turkey and Vegetable Roll-Ups	Nut and Seed Mix or Protein-Packed Strawberry Cheesecake	Baked Cod with Lemon and Dill

Week 3: Advanced Techniques and Diverse Recipes

As you start the third week of your carb-cycling journey, you have a better understanding of the fundamentals and have made the required adjustments based on your body's input. To keep things interesting and challenging, apply some advanced techniques and diversify your recipes.

This week, you'll learn about the significance of meal scheduling and how it affects your metabolism and energy levels. Consuming carbs, for example, before and after a workout can help fuel your exercise and aid in recovery. You will also learn about the advantages of intermittent fasting and how to include it into your carb-cycling strategy.

This week will also introduce you to a selection of new meals that are not only delicious but also in line with your carb-cycling aims. To avoid boredom and to ensure that you are getting a well-rounded array of nutrients, it is critical to have a varied range of recipes in your arsenal. These recipes, ranging from savory foods to sweet sweets, will demonstrate that eating healthy does not have to be dull or uninteresting.

Remember that the key to carb cycling success is consistency and listening to your body. It's fine to make adjustments as needed, and it's critical to be kind with yourself. This is a journey, not a race, and having ups and downs is normal. Maintain your commitment, remain optimistic, and don't be scared to attempt new things. You're doing fantastic, and this week will bring new difficulties and potential for advancement. Accept them with a cheerful attitude and an open mind.

Day	Breakfast	Lunch	Snack	Dinner
15	Berry and Yogurt Parfait	Chickpea and Vegetable Curry	Trail Mix or Protein-Packed Chocolate Cake	Pasta with Roasted Vegetables
16	Avocado and Egg Toast	Pasta with Tomato and Basil Sauce	Fruit and Nut Bars or Protein-Packed Vanilla Ice Cream	Vegetable and Lentil Curry
17	Banana and Nut Muffins	Brown Rice and Bean Bowl	Oatmeal and Raisin Energy Bites or Baked Apple with Cinnamon	Pasta with Roasted Vegetables and Pesto
18	Almond Flour Pancakes	Beef and Vegetable Salad	Apple and Almond Butter Sandwich or Chocolate and Banana Mug Cake	Lemon Garlic Roasted Chicken
19	Chia Seed Pudding	Shrimp and Vegetable Skewers	Berry and Banana Smoothie or Berry and Yogurt Parfait	Baked Salmon with Asparagus
20	Flaxseed Muffins	Tuna and	Peanut Butter and Jelly Energy	Beef Stir-Fry with

Day	Breakfast	Lunch	Snack	Dinner
		Cucumber Roll-Ups	Bites or Oatmeal and Peanut Butter Cookies	Broccoli
21	Egg and Sausage Breakfast Burrito	Chicken and Cheese Lettuce Wraps	Chocolate and Banana Smoothie or Pineapple and Coconut Sorbet	Pork Chops with Roasted Vegetables

Week 4: Solidifying Habits and Preparing for Continuation

As you enter the final week of your 4-week carb-cycling meal plan, it's time to reflect on your progress, cement the habits you've established, and plan for the next phase of your journey. This week is all about reinforcing your positive improvements and positioning yourself for long-term success.

You should have a basic understanding of how carb cycling works, how your body reacts to varied carbohydrate consumption amounts, and how to plan and prepare meals that correspond with your goals. You've also learned the value of meal planning, the advantages of intermittent fasting, and have added several new recipes to your repertoire.

Focus on consistency and awareness this week. Pay attention to how you feel, both physically and mentally, and change your approach as needed. Remember that carb cycling is a flexible technique that must be tailored to your own needs.

Take some time this week to plan for the future as well. Consider your goals and how carb cycling can help you achieve them in the future. Consider any obstacles you may face and devise a strategy to overcome them. Carb cycling can be a crucial tool in your arsenal, whether your aim is weight loss, muscle gain, or simply maintaining a healthy lifestyle.

As you progress, remember that the road to optimal health and wellness is a marathon, not a sprint. It is normal to experience setbacks, and it is critical to remain flexible and adaptable. Maintain your commitment to your goals, remain optimistic, and remember to enjoy the process. You can do it!

Day	Breakfast	Lunch	Snack	Dinner
22	Mango and Coconut Smoothie	Quinoa and Vegetable Salad	Cucumber and Hummus Roll-Ups or Apple and Cinnamon Muffins	Creamy Pumpkin Soup
23	Apple and Cinnamon Oatmeal	Vegetable and Lentil Soup	Almond and Coconut Energy Bites or Berry Protein Gelato	Vegetable Minestrone
24	Peanut Butter and Banana Pancakes	Chickpea and Tomato Stew	Avocado and Tomato Salsa or Protein Chocolate Pudding	Vegetable and Tofu Stir-Fry
25	Smoked Salmon and Cream Cheese Omelette	Turkey and Avocado Salad	Berry and Chia Seed Pudding or Protein Cheesecake Bites	Zucchini Noodles with Pesto and Cherry Tomatoes
26	Almond and Berry Smoothie	Chicken and Avocado Salad	Cheese and Vegetable Sticks or Protein Chocolate Chip Cookies	Baked Cod with Lemon and Dill
27	Avocado and Tomato Salad	Beef and Mushroom	Chocolate and Almond Smoothie or Protein Lemon	Chicken Fajitas with Bell Peppers and Onions

Day	Breakfast	Lunch	Snack	Dinner
		Skewers	Bars	
28	Turkey and Avocado Wrap	Grilled Chicken Salad	Nut and Seed Mix or Protein-Packed Peanut Butter Cups	Grilled Shrimp with Garlic and Herbs

Conclusion

Reflecting on the Carb-Cycling Journey

A carb-cycling path needs effort, strategy, and a willingness to adapt. It is more than just a nutritional change; it is a lifestyle shift. As you near the end of this course, it is critical to reflect on the information you have learned, the progress you have made, and the problems you have faced.

Key Takeaways:

Understanding the Fundamentals: Carb-cycling may appear intimidating at first, but as you read farther into the guide, you realized its essential concepts, benefits, and adaptability to your personal requirements and goals. You discovered that it is a flexible procedure rather than a rigid, one-size-fits-all approach.

Meal Preparation and Planning: You learned that choosing proper foods, portion sizes, and aligning meals with high-carb and low-carb days are critical to carb-cycling success. You also learned about macronutrient balance, nutritional timing, clever ingredient substitutions, batch cooking, and meal preservation.

Adapting Carbohydrate Cycling to Your Goals: The guide taught you how to adjust carb-cycling to your personal goals, whether they were weight loss, muscle gain, sports performance, or addressing the demands of specific groups such as vegetarians or elderly.

Combining Carb-Cycling and Exercise: Exercise is essential for a healthy lifestyle and successful carb-cycling. You learned about exercise science, workout scheduling, the value of rest and recuperation, and how to deal with common issues like energy slumps and cravings.

Reading about other people's successes and problems gave motivation, insights, and a sense of camaraderie.

Common Problems and Troubleshooting: Even with meticulous planning, setbacks are unavoidable. You studied how to deal with food-related issues such as cost, time, and ingredient availability, as well as social and lifestyle issues such as eating out, going to social gatherings, and traveling.

Advanced Carb-Cycling tactics: As your confidence built, you may have experimented with advanced tactics such as combining carb-cycling with intermittent fasting, ketosis, or adapting for different types of activity.

Reflecting on Your Experience:

As you finish this book, take some time to reflect on your accomplishments, new habits, and positive changes in your body and mind. Describe any difficulties you experienced and how you overcome them. This reflection will give you useful insights into what worked well, what didn't, and what you might modify or improve in the future.

A Look Ahead:

Completing this guide is a huge accomplishment, but your carb-cycling adventure is far from over. It entails ongoing learning, modifying, and optimizing to meet changing demands and goals. You could want to try out new tactics, tweak your eating plan, or alter your workout program. Remember to be gentle with yourself, to recognize your accomplishments, and to see obstacles as chances for growth and learning.

Embracing a Lifestyle, Not Just a Diet

Carb-cycling is a journey that goes beyond the boundaries of a diet. It is a comprehensive approach to health and wellbeing that includes all elements of our life, from the food we eat to how we exercise, manage stress, and maintain social connections. Adopting carb-cycling as a lifestyle requires a mindset that promotes self-care, mindfulness, and a balanced way of life.

One of the most important components of adopting carb-cycling as a lifestyle is recognizing its adaptability. Carb-cycling is a flexible method that may be adapted to individual needs, tastes, and goals, as opposed to restrictive diets that impose harsh rules and restrictions. It enables for carbohydrate consumption to be varied based on activity levels, energy requirements, and personal goals. Because of its adaptability, it is a sustainable method that can be incorporated into daily life without generating undue stress or deprivation.

The emphasis on complete, nutrient-dense foods is another crucial part of adopting carb-cycling as a lifestyle. Carb-cycling emphasizes the eating of entire grains, lean proteins, healthy fats, and a variety of fruits and vegetables rather than relying on processed foods or quick solutions. This not only gives the body the nutrition it needs to function properly, but it also encourages a healthy connection with food. It promotes mindful eating, awareness of hunger and fullness cues, and an emphasis on nourishing rather than restricting the body.

In addition to dietary adjustments, adopting carb-cycling as a lifestyle requires frequent physical activity. Exercise is an essential component of any healthy lifestyle and is critical to the success of a carb-cycling regimen. Regular physical activity aids in blood sugar regulation, insulin sensitivity, muscle mass gain, and overall fitness. Endorphins, or 'feel-good' hormones, are also released, which can help to alleviate stress and boost mood.

Adopting carb-cycling as a lifestyle also entails being aware of stress and its effects on the body. Chronic stress can cause a variety of health issues, such as weight gain, insulin resistance, and an increased risk of chronic diseases. It is critical to identify effective stress management techniques, whether through mindfulness practices, deep breathing exercises, spending time in nature, or engaging in activities that provide joy and relaxation.

Finally, adopting carb-cycling as a lifestyle necessitates an appreciation for the value of social ties and support. Starting a carb-cycling journey can be difficult, and having a support network of friends, family, or a community of like-minded people can make all the difference. Sharing experiences, trading insights and recipes, and providing support and accountability can all contribute to a more enjoyable and sustainable journey.

It is about making informed decisions, being aware of our bodies, and taking a long-term approach to health and fitness. Recognizing the flexibility of carbohydrate cycling, focusing on complete, nutrient-dense diets, adding regular physical activity, reducing stress, and maintaining social ties and support are all important. By adopting carb-cycling as a way of life rather than merely a diet, we can make a good and long-term adjustment in our lives that promotes general well-being, both physically and psychologically.

Appendices

Glossary of Terms and Concepts

Glossary for Chapter 1: The Comprehensive Guide to Carbohydrates

Carbohydrates: Organic compounds consisting of carbon, hydrogen, and oxygen, which are a primary source of energy for the body.

Simple Carbs: Carbohydrates that are quickly digested and absorbed, leading to rapid spikes in blood sugar. Examples include sugars found in candies, baked goods, and many processed foods.

Complex Carbs: Carbohydrates that are broken down and absorbed more slowly, providing sustained energy. They are typically found in whole grains, legumes, and vegetables.

Glucose: A simple sugar that is an important energy source in living organisms and is a component of many carbohydrates.

Glycogen: A storage form of glucose, primarily found in the liver and muscles.

Insulin: A hormone produced in the pancreas that regulates the amount of glucose in the blood.

Fiber: A type of carbohydrate that the body can't digest. It moves through the body undigested, keeping the digestive system clean and healthy.

Blood Sugar: The concentration of glucose present in the blood.

Nutrient-Dense: Foods that are high in nutrients but relatively low in calories, providing a rich supply of vitamins, minerals, and other essential substances relative to their caloric content.

Glossary for Chapter 2: Diving Deep into Carb-Cycling

Carb-Cycling: A dietary approach that alternates between high and low carbohydrate intake days.

Metabolic Flexibility: The body's ability to switch between burning carbohydrates and fats for energy.

Ketones: Organic compounds produced in the liver, especially during periods of low carbohydrate intake, used as an alternative energy source.

Insulin: A hormone responsible for regulating blood sugar levels by facilitating the uptake of glucose into cells.

GABA (Gamma-Aminobutyric Acid): A neurotransmitter that plays a key role in mood regulation and has a calming effect on the nervous system.

Neurotransmitter: Chemical messengers that transmit signals in the brain.

Brain Fog: A state of mental confusion or lack of clarity.

Neurocognitive Function: Pertains to the mental processes of perception, memory, judgment, and reasoning.

Glossary of Chapter 3: The Mechanics of Carb-Cycling

Carb-Cycling: A dietary approach where carbohydrate intake fluctuates between high and low on different days.

Metabolic Rate: The rate at which the body expends energy or burns calories.

Glycogen: A form of glucose storage in the body, primarily found in the liver and muscles.

Anabolic Window: A post-workout period where the body is primed to absorb nutrients for recovery.

Sedentary: A lifestyle with only minimal physical activity, typically associated with desk jobs or prolonged sitting.

Proteins: Essential macronutrients responsible for building and repairing tissues.

Fats: Macronutrients that provide energy, support cell growth, and regulate hormones.

Carb Timing: The strategic intake of carbohydrates at specific times to optimize metabolic responses and energy levels.

Glossary for Chapter 4: Overcoming Weight and Fitness Plateaus

Plateau: A phase in a fitness journey where progress, be it weight loss or muscle gain, seems to halt despite consistent efforts.

Adaptive Mechanisms: The body's inherent ability to adjust and respond to various stimuli, leading to changes in metabolism and other physiological processes.

Carb Refeed: A deliberate, significant increase in carb intake, designed to jolt the metabolism and break through plateaus.

Fat Metabolism: The process by which the body breaks down stored fat to produce energy.

Macronutrients: The primary nutrients our body needs in large amounts, namely carbohydrates, proteins, and fats.

Caloric Intake: The total number of calories consumed in a day, influencing weight loss, maintenance, or gain.

Fat Reserves: Stored fat in the body, which can be used as an energy source during periods of caloric deficit or low carbohydrate intake.

Glossary for Chapter 5: Mastering Meal Planning and Prep

Batch Cooking: A method of preparing large quantities of meals at once, intended for consumption over several days or weeks.

Airtight Containers: Storage containers that are sealed completely, preventing the entry or exit of air, thus keeping food fresh for longer.

Parboiling: Partially cooking food by boiling, which can then be finished by another method like roasting or sautéing.

Carb-Cycling Menu: A planned set of meals that align with the high-carb and low-carb days of the carb-cycling schedule.

Ingredient Swaps: Replacing one ingredient in a recipe with another to align with dietary requirements or preferences.

Labeling: Clearly marking storage containers with details about the contents and date of preparation.

Thawing: The process of allowing frozen food to return to a normal state, usually by placing it in the refrigerator.

Kitchen Hacks: Innovative and efficient techniques or methods to simplify cooking or meal preparation.

Glossary for Chapter 7: Personalizing Carb-Cycling for Your Goals

Hypertrophy: Scientific term for muscle growth.

Glycogen: Stored form of carbohydrates in the muscles and liver, used as a primary energy source during high-intensity activities.

Cortisol: A hormone, often referred to as the 'stress hormone', that can influence muscle breakdown and recovery.

Insulin: A hormone that regulates blood sugar levels and plays a role in nutrient uptake by muscles.

Veganism: A dietary and lifestyle choice that excludes all animal products.

Metabolic Rate: The rate at which the body expends energy or burns calories.

Protein Synthesis: The process by which the body produces new proteins, essential for muscle repair and growth.

Nutrient Deficiency: A state where the body lacks essential nutrients, which can impact health and well-being.

Bone Density: A measure of bone health, indicating strength and risk for conditions like osteoporosis.

Plant-based Proteins: Protein sources derived from plants, including lentils, chickpeas, tofu, and more.

Glossary for Chapter 8: Synergizing Carb-Cycling with Workouts

Carb-Cycling: A dietary approach where one alternates between high and low carbohydrate intake days to maximize fat burning and muscle growth.

Glycogen: A form of glucose storage in the body, primarily found in the liver and muscles. Used as a primary energy source during high-intensity workouts.

Micro-tears: Small tears in muscle fibers resulting from intense physical activity, leading to muscle growth when repaired.

Recovery: The process of restoring health and strength, both mentally and physically, after physical exertion.

Rest Days: Scheduled days off from intense workouts, allowing the body and mind to heal and rejuvenate.

Hormonal Balance: The equilibrium of various hormones in the body, crucial for numerous bodily functions, including metabolism, mood regulation, and tissue function.

Inflammation: A natural response of the body to injury or harmful stimuli, often resulting in pain, redness, heat, and swelling.

Post-workout: The period immediately following a workout session, critical for recovery and muscle growth.

Glossary for Chapter 9: Real-Life Journeys: Success Stories and Lessons

Carb-Cycling: A dietary approach where one

alternates between high and low carbohydrate intake days.

Motivation: The drive or reason for acting or behaving in a particular way.

Resilience: The capacity to recover quickly from difficulties; toughness.

Adaptability: The ability to adjust to new conditions.

Potluck Dinners: A gathering where each guest contributes a different, often homemade, dish of food to be shared.

No-Cook Recipes: Dishes that require no cooking and can be prepared using raw ingredients.

Overnight Oats: A breakfast dish made by soaking rolled oats in liquid (like milk or yogurt) overnight.

Journaling: The practice of keeping a diary or journal that explores thoughts and feelings surrounding the events of one's life.

Stepping Stones: A circumstance or action that helps one to make progress towards a goal.

Glossary for Chapter 10: Troubleshooting and Common Concerns

Energy Slumps: Periods of pronounced fatigue or decreased energy, often experienced during dietary changes.

Cravings: A powerful desire for specific foods, which can be driven by both physical hunger and emotional triggers.

Mindset: An individual's mental attitude or disposition, which can influence their response to situations.

Growth Mindset: A belief that abilities and intelligence can be developed through dedication and hard work.

Macronutrients: The main nutrients required by the body in large amounts, including carbohydrates, proteins, and fats.

Nutrient-dense Foods: Foods that are high in nutrients but relatively low in calories, providing maximum nutrition with minimal calorie intake.

Support Groups: Communities or gatherings of individuals who provide emotional and moral support for shared challenges or experiences.

Glossary for Chapter 11: Advanced Carb-Cycling Strategies

Aerobic Metabolism: A type of energy production that uses oxygen to convert carbohydrates and fats into energy. It is the primary source of energy during prolonged, moderate-intensity exercise.

Anaerobic Metabolism: A type of energy production that does not require oxygen and uses carbohydrates as the primary source of energy. It is the primary source of energy during short bursts of high-intensity exercise.

Glycogen: The stored form of carbohydrates in the muscles and liver. It is used as a source of energy during exercise.

Intermittent Fasting: A dietary approach that involves alternating between periods of fasting and eating. It has been shown to have potential benefits for weight loss, metabolic health, and overall well-being.

Ketosis: A metabolic state in which the body burns fat for fuel instead of carbohydrates. It can be induced by following a ketogenic diet, which is a low-carb, high-fat diet.

Macronutrients: The three main nutrients that provide energy: carbohydrates, proteins, and fats.

Metabolism: The process by which your body converts food and drink into energy.

Carbohydrate Intake: The amount of carbohydrates consumed in the diet. It can be manipulated in a carb-cycling plan to optimize the body's metabolic response.

Glossary for Conclusion

Carb-Cycling: A dietary approach that involves alternating between high-carb and low-carb days to optimize carbohydrate intake and support various fitness goals.

Mindful Eating: Being fully present and aware during meals, paying attention to hunger and fullness cues, and focusing on nourishing the body rather than restricting it.

Insulin Sensitivity: The ability of the body's cells to respond to insulin, a hormone that regulates blood sugar levels.

Endorphins: Hormones released during exercise that act as natural painkillers and mood elevators.

Insulin Resistance: A condition in which the body's cells do not respond well to insulin, leading to higher levels of insulin in the blood.

Nutrient-Dense Foods: Foods that are high in nutrients but relatively low in calories, such as fruits, vegetables, lean proteins, and whole grains.

Additional Resources: Books, Podcasts, and Websites

Beginning a path toward a better lifestyle may be both gratifying and challenging, especially when you are just getting started. The carb cycling diet is an excellent option for anyone trying to lose weight, increase sports performance, or simply live a healthier lifestyle. As a beginning, though, it is natural to seek assistance and help to ensure you are on the correct course. While this book gives a thorough overview to carb cycling, including tasty recipes to get you started, there are numerous other resources available to supplement your journey. There is a variety of information available to assist you navigate the world of carb cycling, from books and podcasts to websites.

Books are an excellent resource for individuals interested in learning more about carb cycling. Dr. Roman Malkov's book "The Carb Cycling Diet: Balancing High Carb, Low Carb, and No Carb Days for Healthy Weight Loss" comes highly recommended. This book is a comprehensive explanation to carb cycling, explaining the theory and offering practical guidance on how to incorporate it into your daily life. Laura Herring's "Carb Cycling for Beginners: Recipes and Exercises to Lose Weight and Build Muscle" is another fantastic book. This book is ideal for beginners because it includes simple meals and fitness regimens to get you started on your carb cycling journey.

Podcasts are another excellent way to learn while on the road. Amber Wentworth's "The Carb Cycling Podcast" is an excellent resource for anyone interested in carb cycling. Amber discusses her personal carb cycling experiences, interviews experts in the industry, and offers listeners practical suggestions and advice. Dr. Bret Scher's "The Diet Doctor Podcast" is another useful podcast. While this podcast covers a wide range of low carb and ketogenic diet issues, there are numerous episodes dedicated to carb cycling that are well worth listening to.

Websites are also an excellent resource for anyone interested in learning more about carb cycling. Diet Doctor (dietdoctor.com) offers a wealth of information on low carb and ketogenic diets, with a section on carb cycling. You'll find articles, meal plans, and recipes to help you along the way. Bodybuilding.com is another resource. This website contains a variety of information about carb cycling, including how-to articles, food planning, and exercise routines. MyFitnessPal is also a fantastic app for tracking your meals and exercise, which can be very handy when following a carb cycling diet.

There is a variety of material accessible to help you achieve whether you want to read books, listen to podcasts, or browse websites. Finally, like with any diet or fitness routine, consistency and perseverance are the keys to success with carb cycling. By arming yourself with the necessary knowledge and tools, you will be well on your way to accomplishing your health and fitness objectives.

Index of Recipes by Carb Count and Dietary Restrictions

Low Carb and Keto-Friendly:

Almond Flour Pancakes
Chia Seed Pudding
Coconut Flour Waffles
Smoked Salmon and Cream Cheese Omelette
Almond and Berry Smoothie
Avocado and Tomato Salad
Chicken and Vegetable Stir-Fry
Turkey and Cheese Roll-Ups
Egg and Sausage Breakfast Burrito
Almond and Coconut Granola
Bacon and Egg Breakfast Cups
Spinach and Feta Omelette
Turkey and Avocado Wrap
Grilled Chicken Salad
Shrimp and Avocado Salad
Beef and Broccoli Stir-Fry
Chicken and Vegetable Skewers
Tuna Salad Stuffed Avocado
Egg Salad Lettuce Wraps
Turkey and Vegetable Roll-Ups
Chicken and Avocado Salad
Beef and Vegetable Salad
Shrimp and Vegetable Skewers
Tuna and Cucumber Roll-Ups
Chicken and Cheese Lettuce Wraps
Beef and Mushroom Skewers
Turkey and Avocado Salad
Zucchini Noodles with Pesto and Cherry
Tomatoes
Lemon Garlic Roasted Chicken
Baked Salmon with Asparagus
Beef Stir-Fry with Broccoli
Pork Chops with Green Beans
Shrimp Scampi with Zucchini Noodles
Grilled Steak with Roasted Vegetables
Baked Cod with Lemon and Dill
Chicken Fajitas with Bell Peppers and Onions
Pork Tenderloin with Roasted Brussels Sprouts
Grilled Shrimp with Garlic and Herbs
Beef and Vegetable Kebabs
Chicken and Vegetable Stir-Fry
Pork Chops with Roasted Vegetables
Baked Tilapia with Lemon and Herbs
Beef and Mushroom Stir-Fry
Chicken and Asparagus Stir-Fry
Spicy Shrimp and Cauliflower Rice
Cucumber and Hummus Roll-Ups
Almond and Coconut Energy Bites

Avocado and Tomato Salsa
Berry and Chia Seed Pudding
Cheese and Vegetable Sticks
Chocolate and Almond Smoothie
Nut and Seed Mix
Berry Protein Gelato
Protein Chocolate Pudding
Protein Cheesecake Bites
Protein Chocolate Chip Cookies
Protein Lemon Bars
Protein-Packed Peanut Butter Cups
Protein-Packed Strawberry Cheesecake
Protein-Packed Chocolate Cake
Protein-Packed Vanilla Ice Cream

Moderate Carbs:

Quinoa and Vegetable Breakfast Bowl
Sweet Potato and Black Bean Hash
Peanut Butter and Banana Smoothie
Apple and Cinnamon Porridge
Berry and Yogurt Parfait
Avocado and Egg Toast
Banana and Nut Muffins
Chocolate and Peanut Butter Smoothie
Apple and Cinnamon Oatmeal
Berry and Nut Smoothie
Peanut Butter and Banana Pancakes
Mango and Coconut Smoothie
Scrambled Eggs with Spinach and Feta
Chickpea and Vegetable Stir-Fry
Quinoa and Black Bean Salad
Sweet Potato and Lentil Curry
Brown Rice and Vegetable Bowl
Pasta Primavera
Vegetable and Bean Burrito
Lentil and Vegetable Stew
Vegetable and Quinoa Stir-Fry
Chickpea and Vegetable Curry
Pasta with Tomato and Basil Sauce
Brown Rice and Bean Bowl
Vegetable and Lentil Soup
Quinoa and Vegetable Salad
Chickpea and Tomato Stew
Pasta with Vegetable and Bean Sauce
Spaghetti Squash with Tomato Sauce and
Parmesan
Lentil and Vegetable Stuffed Bell Peppers
Sweet Potato and Chickpea Curry

Vegetable and Bean Pasta
Quinoa and Vegetable Stir-Fry
Chickpea and Tomato Stew
Pasta with Vegetable and Bean Sauce
Brown Rice and Bean Bowl
Vegetable and Lentil Soup
Quinoa and Vegetable Salad
Creamy Pumpkin Soup
Vegetable Minestrone
Vegetable and Tofu Stir-Fry
Pasta with Roasted Vegetables
Vegetable and Lentil Curry
Pasta with Roasted Vegetables and Pesto
Apple and Almond Butter Sandwich
Berry and Banana Smoothie

Peanut Butter and Jelly Energy Bites
Chocolate and Banana Smoothie
Trail Mix
Fruit and Nut Bars
Oatmeal and Raisin Energy Bites
Baked Apple with Cinnamon
Chocolate and Banana Mug Cake
Berry and Yogurt Parfait
Oatmeal and Peanut Butter Cookies
Pineapple and Coconut Sorbet
Chocolate and Avocado Mousse
Apple and Cinnamon Muffins
Banana Berry Oatmeal
Whole Grain Pancakes with Apple and Nuts

Measurement And Conversion Table

Volume

Measurement	Equals	Also Equals
1 c.	8 fluid ounces	237 milliliters
1 pint (2 c.s)	16 fluid ounces	473 milliliters
1 quart (2 pints)	32 fluid ounces	946 milliliters
1 gallon (4 quarts)	128 fluid ounces	3.785 liters

Weight

Measurement	Equals	Also Equals
1 ounce	1/16 pound	28.35 grams
1 pound	16 ounces	453.59 grams

Cooking Measures

Measurement	Equals	Also Equals
1 Tbsp.	3 Tsp..s	15 milliliters
1 c.	16 Tbsp.s	237 milliliters
1 fluid ounce	2 Tbsp.s	29.57 milliliters

Oven Temperatures:

Measurement Fahrenheit	Equals Celsius
225°F	110°C
250°F	130°C
275°F	140°C
300°F	150°C
325°F	165°C
350°F	180°C
375°F	190°C
400°F	200°C
425°F	220°C
450°F	230°C
475°F	245°C
500°F	260°C

Dry Measures:

Measurement	Equals	Also Equals
1 ounce	28.35 grams	
1 pound	16 ounces	453.59 grams

Made in the USA
Las Vegas, NV
03 March 2024

86658750R00063